WHERE DID HOWDY GO?

Ruth C. Weidman & John E. Becker

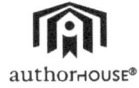

authorHOUSE®

AuthorHouse™
1663 Liberty Drive
Bloomington, IN 47403
www.authorhouse.com
Phone: 1-800-839-8640

First published by AuthorHouse   2/3/2010

ISBN: 978-1-4490-5879-1 (e)
ISBN: 978-1-4490-5878-4 (sc)

Library of Congress Control Number: 2009913264

Printed in the United States of America
Bloomington, Indiana

This book is printed on acid-free paper.

Dedicated to the loving memory of Rusty and Howdy

PREFACE

Howdy and I fell in love, and the depth of that love never changed in all our years together. If ever two people were meant for each other, we were that couple.

There was never any doubt, suspicion, or mistrust. I believe, with all my heart, we were destined to be together, and that God blessed us with a boundless love few couples ever experience.

In Howdy's eyes, I could do no wrong. I remember my mother saying that I could tell Howdy in broad daylight that it was the dark of night, and he would've believed me. According to her, it wasn't supposed to be like that. But I loved it!

There was an eleven-and-a-half year difference in our ages, and my mother had grave doubts that we could overcome such an obstacle. Several times she asked me what I wanted with a man that much older than myself. I could only tell her that it seemed like there wasn't an age difference at all - we thought completely alike about everything.

Of course, no one ever suspected that the difference in our ages would make it possible for me to take care of Howdy in the last years of his life.

Looking back on it now, I understand that caring for Howdy was the principal reason for my being on this earth. In the pages that follow, I'll relate some of the wonderful memories I have of the idyllic romance that Howdy and I shared, and how the terrible disease known as Alzheimer's ended our beautiful dream.

I tried to remember to write down the events of each day of our lives as we went along. But every once in a while, I was either just too tired, or depressed, to take the time to keep up with my notes. Now, I'm really sorry, because I can't remember some of the things that went on during Howdy's illness. But I've tried to reminisce, and that helps to bring back a lot of memories. Most of those memories were good, and some of them were bad, but I've recalled all that I can remember.

Ruth C. Weidman

CHAPTER 1 - FORGETFULLNESS

When I reflect on it now, I can see that the occasional lapses of memory Howdy began experiencing in 1979 were the start of a devastating sequence of events. We had no way of knowing then that it would be the beginning of a terrible nightmare.

Before Howdy's 69th birthday, on March 3, 1979, he seemed to be more and more forgetful. I found myself saying to him all too often, "Boy, you can sure tell you're going to be 69 on your birthday. It's a good thing your head's attached, or you'd forget that, too." He'd look at me with those big, sad-looking, brown eyes, and then we'd both laugh.

A few weeks after Howdy's birthday that year, we went to see my sister, Mary Jane, and her family in Aliquippa, Pennsylvania. During our visit, Mary Jane pointed out how my teasing seemed to hurt Howdy's feelings.

"You ought to stop making those comments about Howdy's forgetfulness," she said. "I think it's really bothering him. Even though you're laughing when you say it, he gets a hurt look on his face."

Occasionally, we need someone to tell us when we're doing something wrong. That was certainly one of those times. Thereafter, I became more aware of Howdy's feelings, and I tried hard not to offend him anymore. But as time went on, I caught myself saying things that upset him, and I found myself saying, "I'm sorry," more and more often. Eventually, the apologies came so frequently that the tears inevitably came, too. It was like someone opening up the floodgates. Sometimes I'd cry on and off for days and days. The pain, borne out of a sense of guilt and frustration, became overwhelming. Many times, I thought my heart would literally break.

I cried more, over a ten-year period, than most people cry in a lifetime. I sometimes wondered where all the tears came from, and why my eyes didn't shrivel up. I also wondered what kept me from just totally breaking down. I cried just as much at the end, as I did in the beginning. It was a good thing

Howdy never lost the ability to express his feelings through facial expressions, and with his eyes. By understanding his bewilderment, yet seeing that loving tenderness in those eyes, I managed to keep going through the darkest days.

From the onset of Howdy's forgetfulness in 1979, until May of 1983, we lived a relatively normal life, without any major incidents. As each year passed, Howdy developed an increasing dislike for the cold winters of the North. Finally, he convinced me we should head for the warmth of the South, and we moved from Ohio to Dade City, Florida, in March of 1981. The decision to go wasn't an easy one, however, as our son, John, and his family, lived in Ohio. I knew we wouldn't see our grandchildren very often, but I was convinced moving would be the best thing for Howdy.

We lived in Florida year-round until 1986. That year we bought a house trailer back in Ohio. For the next few years, we lived six months of the year in our home in Florida, and six months in our home in Ohio. We migrated with the seasons - just like the birds.

Howdy slept a great deal of the time during those long, twenty-one hour, drives between Ohio and Florida. That gave me many hours to reflect on happier times, and I often thought of how Howdy and I met. Looking back, it seemed as if our meeting had been scripted by fate.

CHAPTER 2 - HOW IT ALL BEGAN

In 1941, I moved with my family from our hometown of Pittsburgh, Pennsylvania to Detroit, Michigan. Mary Jane and I found jobs working in factories that made components for military aircraft. We lived with our mother and my son, John, in a small, cramped apartment. I was a riveter and Mary Jane was a welder. We worked long, hard hours with few breaks, but were grateful to have jobs after the lean years of the Depression. Even though we made pretty good money, we hated living in Detroit and longed for the familiar, hilly terrain of home. So, one day early in 1944, we quit our jobs, packed up, and headed home to Pittsburgh.

Our first priority, of course, was finding jobs. Since neither Mary Jane, nor I, drove, or owned a car, we considered ourselves extremely lucky when we both found work at a bakery located just a short streetcar ride from home.

We worked the night shift with a terrific group of girls and a few men. We had a wonderful foreman named Howard. Everyone called him Howdy, and all the girls adored him because he was always smiling, or singing. It didn't take very long for me to understand why the girls were so crazy about Howdy. Not only was he very good-natured, but he also had a heart of gold. I'd never encountered such a caring, sensitive man before. Almost from the beginning, like the other girls, I had a crush on Howdy, and soon I found myself falling in love with him. Of course, I was sure he didn't know I existed.

I worked at the bakery for just a few months when a man working on the oven went into the service, and they needed to train someone to take over his job. I was surprised to find out I'd been selected, and when I learned Howdy would be teaching me how to operate the oven, I was thrilled.

The very first night of my training, Howdy carefully explained the mechanical operation of the oven, the safety precautions, and how to handle the various items that would be baked in the oven. At first, the prospect of being responsible for running such a huge and important piece of equipment was a bit overwhelming. The oven itself was as large as a small room, and if something went wrong with it, a major portion of the bakery operation would be shut down. As you might imagine, I was very intimidated, but Howdy was so patient and encouraging that my mind was soon at ease.

When Howdy finished going over all my responsibilities and answering my questions at the front of the oven, he took me to the back to show me how it fired up. He also showed me how the chain drive worked to move large trays weighing several hundred pounds each. I must have been feeling more comfortable because, as Howdy continued his instruction, I found myself looking at him out of the corner of my eye. Little did I know at the time, but Howdy was doing the same.

Not long after that, we discovered just how strongly we were attracted to each other, and eventually, we began seeing each other. From the very beginning of our relationship, Howdy was the best thing that ever happened to me.

Working at the bakery was more like a family get-together than a job, because we were all so compatible and enjoyed working together. Someone always seemed to be singing, and we laughed a lot. Most of the girls were Italian and wonderful cooks, so occasionally, we'd bring in the makings for an Italian dinner. What wonderful times we had, and we were eating like royalty! We didn't have to worry about the dough for bread or pasta – it was right there at our fingertips.

During those weeks and months, I discovered, for the first time in my life, how it felt to really be in love. And I was as sure of Howdy's love for me as I was of my love for him. The day of our marriage was the happiest day of my life.

Things were great until 1949. We'd moved to Cleveland and our lives seemed ideal. But that year, Howdy suffered a ruptured ulcer and it almost perforated the wall of his stomach. Complicating matters was the fact that I was pregnant at the same time.

For almost two years before his ulcer ruptured, Howdy would occasionally complain about a recurring pain between his shoulder blades in his back. Gradually, the pain became more and more severe. One night, when he came home from work in the middle of the night, he had to crawl up the stairs because the pain was so intense. That's when I insisted on Howdy going to the doctor's the next day. By then, he was so critically ill the doctor insisted on putting him in Doctor's Hospital immediately.

I'd never been around anyone who had an operation before. It was an agonizing ordeal for me as well as Howdy. I waited for nine, excruciating hours, as Howdy lay near death on the operating table. Finally, I was told I could visit him in his room. Nothing could've prepared me for the shock of what I saw. He had a tongue depressor in his mouth, a hose going up his nose, IV's in both arms, a catheter in his penis, and to make things even worse, the next day they put a tube up his rectum - for gas. I still have horrible memories of that gut-wrenching experience. He also had tubes running from his stomach to a tank containing the most terrible looking stuff I ever saw. I was pregnant, so the sight of the liquids in that jar nauseated me, and I wanted to throw up - but I didn't. His private nurse was also pregnant. I never understood how she could deal with all that in her condition.

We lived on one side of town and Doctor's Hospital was located on the opposite side. It took three busses to get to the hospital from our house. I'd go in the morning, then return home when our son, John, got home from school, and both of us would make the trip back. We did that every day until Howdy was allowed to go home. It was exhausting for both John, and me, so we were relieved when it was finally over. But John had an even greater reason for never wanting to see that hospital again, because he had an extremely traumatic experience while Howdy was a patient there.

At that time, children weren't allowed to visit the patients, so I'd leave John in the lobby of the hospital while I went upstairs to visit Howdy. One evening, while I was sitting with Howdy, one of the nurses came down the hall calling for "Mrs. Becker." Since my name was Weidman then, I didn't make the connection immediately. But it finally occurred to me she was looking for me.

When I asked her why she was looking for Mrs. Becker, she said I was needed downstairs in the Emergency Room because a dog had bitten my son. At first, I thought she was joking, but from the urgency in her voice, I could tell she wasn't.

When we arrived in the emergency room, John was crying uncontrollably. It took quite a while for me to settle him down enough for him to tell us what happened. Once he stopped sobbing, he explained how he followed my instructions and stayed in the lobby of the hospital. But shortly after I went upstairs, a woman came rushing into the lobby with a small dog. Since she couldn't take the dog into the hospital with her, she dumped it in John's lap and told him to watch it until she came back. John said that he sat as rigid as a stone for what seemed like hours. I knew that was probably true because John had been bitten by dogs twice before, and he was very nervous around them.

After a long wait, John decided I was late, so he placed the dog on the floor while he went to look for a clock. When he went back and tried to pick the dog up again, it bit him. John began screaming hysterically, and caused quite a stir throughout the hospital. The nurse said she was surprised we didn't hear him screaming up on the fourth floor.

The hospital staff had to call the police, because the law stipulated that dogs guilty of biting someone had to be quarantined for a period of time, so they could be tested for rabies. When the woman who owned the dog found out it would be quarantined, she became very upset. She begged me not to allow them to take her dog away, but according to the police, there was nothing I could do about it. So, the woman became hysterical, and it was quite a scene! I couldn't get over the fact she had the nerve to be mad at us because her dog had to be quarantined. Needless to say, John never watched anyone's dog again after that.

Howdy's recovery went very well. He ate baby food for several weeks, then junior food, before he went back to a normal diet. Once he returned to eating regular food, he never had any more problems.

In July, we had a beautiful baby girl. She had dark hair, a nice round head, and the smoothest skin you could imagine. Of course, we were prejudiced. We named her Barbara Lynn, and Howdy was planning on calling her "Babs." The day after she was born, however, she started turning yellow. By the next day, she was even more yellow, and we were terribly worried. On the third day, the doctor told us there was an RH factor making our baby jaundiced. Because my blood was negative, and Howdy's was positive, the two blood types just didn't go together. The hospital staff seemed to be running around like crazy in a frantic effort to save our baby. Finally, the doctor asked us if we had someone who could donate blood. Howdy asked at the bakery and a young fellow volunteered to donate his.

Unfortunately, by that time, it was hopeless. Barbara Lynn's veins were so small the donated blood went straight into her tissues instead of her veins. When the doctor came into my room and asked me if I wanted her baptized I knew my worst fears were realized. It was the fourth day of her life, and the worst day of ours. As the minutes slowly ticked away, she gradually turned a very deep shade of orange. Within a few hours, she was gone.

"Barbara Lynn Weidman," lived such a short life. To have experienced the joy of carrying her for nine months, and to have dreamed the dreams that mothers do, only to lose her, was devastating. What a terrible tragedy. I'm convinced the doctor should have known by the blood tests we had an RH problem, and should've been prepared for it. I'd never seen Howdy cry before, and he cried helplessly – we all did. We not only felt our own loss, but we also felt sorry for the man who donated the blood, because he thought it was his blood that caused her death. He was deaf, and Howdy couldn't sign, so Howdy had a very difficult time convincing him it wasn't his fault.

Howdy and I never tried to have any more children after that. It was just the three of us from then on, Howdy, John, and me.

That was the first time in my life I was mad at God. It was hard for me to understand why he'd take our precious little girl away from us. I never dreamed that later in my life I'd be mad at God again for allowing the man I loved to suffer and die so terribly. Fortunately, in time, I got over those feelings and regained my faith.

Of course, from that point on, we knew John would be our only child, and Howdy and I certainly thanked God for giving him to us. Howdy accepted my son as his own, and they got along well. When John graduated from high school in 1960, Howdy decided he should go to college. Howdy never had the opportunity to attend college, so he wanted John to have that chance. I wanted him to go into the service, because I felt the discipline and responsibility he'd learn there would make him a better person. But Howdy was adamant, and I allowed him to make the final decision.

CHAPTER 3 – HAPPIER TIMES

Howdy and I both worked. He continued to work as a baker, and I was a cashier in a supermarket. Howdy worked weird hours. Since his specialty was baking bread, and bread was the first thing to be finished in the morning, he generally went in to start work around 4:00 P.M. With him working nights and me working days, we didn't get to spend much time together. When we did get together, we were so glad to see each other that it seemed as if we never had time to argue about anything. When he came home at 3:00 in the morning, I'd be up waiting for him, with a good, hot meal ready as soon as he walked in the door. After cleaning up, we'd go to bed. I had to get up again at 6:00 to go to work, so he'd be gone when I came home - certainly no time for arguing.

A great deal of the time, while we were married, my mother lived with us. For the most part, it worked out well, because she did the everyday cleaning, washing, and cooking. Another fringe benefit of her being with us was she took care of John. Knowing she was watching out for him, while I was at work, made things a lot less stressful for me. No wonder I was able to get up in the middle of the night and take care of Howdy without being too cranky. Actually, I don't know how we'd have gotten by without her. My mother was great! The best part was how well she and Howdy got along. He never really minded having her with us, or at least he never told me he did. All the things she did for us gave us more time to be together on our days off. Howdy always wanted me to be close to him. He never wanted me out of his sight, so I tried not to do work around the house we couldn't do together. Occasionally, we'd go out to dinner at a nice restaurant, but we mainly enjoyed having time to share together at home. I usually spent most of my time doing the heavy chores around the house like scrubbing the floors, washing walls, yard work, and other things my mother was unable to do. It worked out quite well because her days off were on my days off.

Howdy retired in 1972, at the age of 62. At first, he seemed to get along okay. I was still working each day, but he had my mother to talk to, and that seemed to help him get by. Sadly, my mother died the next year. I think Howdy felt her loss even more than I did. He became lonely and depressed after she passed away. It wasn't quite so bad in the spring or summer, when he could putter around in the yard, but he hated winters. Somehow, he managed to endure the loneliness for six more years.

Finally, during the long, icy winter of 1977-78, Howdy couldn't stand it anymore. I remember coming home on one cold and dreary afternoon. When I walked up to the front door, after I put my car in the garage, the door was open and Howdy was standing in the doorway. He looked like the saddest human being I'd ever seen. He was almost in tears, and when I asked him what was wrong, he begged me to retire. He'd become extremely depressed, and he hated being cooped up in the house all day by himself. We really still needed my income, because Howdy's pension from the Baker's Union wasn't that great, but one look at him and I knew I had to retire. So, I promised him I'd quit the next year, and that made him very happy. I officially retired as a cashier for Pick-N-Pay Supermarkets on May 25, 1979, and neither of us ever regretted that decision.

After working for 24 years, and residing a little over twenty years in the city of Brunswick, Ohio, it took me a little while to get into retirement living. Since it was summer, Howdy and I busied ourselves with yard work and fixing things up around the house. I'm not sure when we started talking about it, but before long, we decided to sell the house and move to Delaware, Ohio. John, his wife Betsy, and our two grandchildren, John and Janean, had moved to Delaware, which is about twenty miles north of Columbus, in March of that year. Because our grandson, John Howard, had been born in St. Paul, Minnesota in 1970, and Janean Lynn, our granddaughter, had been born in Florida in 1973, we lamented how seldom we saw them - usually only once, or twice, a year. Since they were settled back in Ohio, it seemed like an ideal time for us to move closer to them, and get to see our grandchildren every day.

It was amazing how much stuff we'd accumulated after living in our house for 21 years. We spent lots of time just going through everything, and getting rid of most of it. I'd like to have a nickel for all the times we said, "What in the world have we been hanging onto this for?"

Going through boxes and boxes of useless items was just one part of getting the house ready to be sold. Cleaning, scrubbing, painting, and fixing things seemed to consume every waking moment. We were determined to enjoy our retirement, so we made sure we left time each week to visit old friends, go out to a restaurant, or go sightseeing someplace. We even went to a couple of plays. Those were really carefree, happy days.

One fond memory of that summer was the time we spent with some of our very best friends. It's a shame, but when you're working, you lose touch with people you were close to at one point or another in your life. So, we made sure we saw as many of those friends as we could, and as it turned out, many of them we never saw again.

It took a while to get the house sold, but finally, by March of 1980, we'd left our home in Brunswick and moved into an apartment in Delaware. It took quite some time for us to get used to the cramped surroundings of a two-bedroom apartment, but being near our son and his family made it bearable. Our original plan was to buy a house in Delaware and spend the rest of our days there. But plans don't always go as you'd like them to, and that was one of those times. We spent a lot of time looking at houses, but never did find anything that appealed to both of us.

Howdy's brother, Herbert, and his wife Sylvia, had retired to Zephyrhills, Florida a few years before we moved to Delaware. They'd been after us for some time to come down and visit them, so we decided to fly down that fall. Herbert said he'd pick us up at the airport, we'd stay with them, and he and Sylvia would drive us around to see some of the sights of Florida.

It's amazing how much we were able to cram into one week. We visited Busch Gardens, Disney World, Citrus Gardens, watched manatees swimming at Homosassa Springs, and even found time to just lounge around in Herbert and Sylvia's yard and talk. The highlight for us was the night we all went to The Kapok Tree Inn in Tampa. Herbert and Sylvia had told us how great it was, and they were right! The place was packed, and we had to wait almost an hour to be seated, but the wait was well worth it. The food was excellent and the service terrific. The setting was truly spectacular with roman columns and statues adorning the building inside and out - we were extremely impressed. It was where I first discovered hush puppies, and they're still the best I ever ate.

While we were down there, Herbert and Sylvia talked us into looking at mobile home parks. I never dreamed we'd ever buy a mobile home; it just seemed like a way to pass the time. But one day, we went to a park in Dade City, which is just a little north of Zephyrhills. When we went into one of the models I couldn't get over how much it was like a real house inside. It was a particularly lovely doublewide with an open kitchen, dining area, huge master bedroom with walk in closets, and a gorgeous terrazzo floored 20 foot x16 foot screened in sun porch. Howdy and I fell in love with the place the minute we walked in the door.

Howdy hardly ever asked for anything for himself, so I was very surprised when he turned to me while we were standing in the sun porch and said, "Buy me this."

It was obvious that Howdy was taken with the place, but I still asked him if he was sure, and he said, "Oh, yes!"

So we put down a deposit and began planning our move to Florida.

I knew how much Howdy hated the cold northern winters, and I knew he was very much in love with the trailer in Dade City, but the thought of leaving our grandchildren after such a short time was extremely difficult for me. When the time finally came to go, I cried and cried.

We moved to Florida in March of 1981. Little could I have imagined that the next few weeks and months would be some of the happiest of my life, only to be followed by the darkest period of my life during which I'd reach the very depths of despair.

From the moment we moved into our beautiful trailer in Dade City we were surrounded by dear friends. Having Herbert and Sylvia in Zephyrhills, just a short drive away was great, and we became closer than ever. They introduced us to all of their friends, and they soon became our good friends, too. Some of our very best friends were Ethel and Jim Smith, Aileen and Chuck Grof, Anna Mae and Walter, the Schmidts, and Dora and Leo Zilla. Then there were our neighbors at Country Aire Manor trailer park. It was as if all of the people in the park were also wonderful friends.

Once we settled into our new home in Florida, we were constantly on the go. There are so many attractions for tourists in Florida, and we wanted to see as many of them as we could. We traveled to the Panhandle and the sparkling white beaches of Panama City. We went down the Gulf Coast from Cedar Key to Fort Myers, and just about everywhere in between. Places like Homosossa Springs, Tarpon Springs, Clearwater Beach, Sarasota, and St. Petersburg were some of our favorite destinations.

My brother, Harry, was retired and divorced and was still living in Michigan. We invited him to spend a few months with us in Florida. We had two bedrooms and two baths, so we had plenty of room. He agreed, and stayed with us about five months that winter (Harry's visit became an annual event every year until we moved back to Ohio again).

He had some of his own things he wanted to bring to Florida. So in October of 1981, Harry and his son, his son's wife, and children came with him when he drove down. Harry's son and his family stayed for a week sightseeing, and had a nice vacation. After they left, Harry stayed on.

For the next couple of months we really had a good time, all three of us. By then, Howdy and I had seen quite a bit of Florida, but even with all of the sightseeing we did in that first year, I don't think we saw a tenth of it.

Harry was very interested in space exploration, so one of the first places we visited, while he stayed with us, was the John F. Kennedy Space Center and Cape Canaveral. The crowds there made me very uncomfortable, but crowds didn't bother Howdy and Harry, so I went along with them. Although I really enjoyed seeing the space center and learning about our space program, I was always happy to get back home. If we could've somehow arranged to just have the three of us visit those places by ourselves, I'd have been much happier. Fortunately, Howdy was still in relatively good health at that time, so I'm pleased he got to see those attractions before he became too ill to enjoy them.

We also got down to the Everglades, which was a wonderful experience for all of us. Traveling put a lot of miles on the car, so we were fortunate our car was still in pretty good shape.

One of the trips Howdy really enjoyed was the day we spent at Bok Gardens. There is a bell tower at the gardens, and because Howdy loved music, the ringing of the bells, with their melodic tones, impressed him. In fact, he didn't want to leave when it was time to go. To please him we stayed an extra hour. I'm glad we saw as many tourist attractions as we did early in our time in Florida.

Another one of Howdy's favorite spots was the Ringling Brothers Museum in Sarasota. Because we were fortunate enough to live in a good, central location in Florida, a lot of the places we were able to visit in one day, which was a lot easier on all of us.

Howdy's sister, Ruth, also paid us a visit shortly after we moved to Florida. She was retired by then and finally had the time to travel, which she dearly loved to do. We took her to see a woman she'd worked with who'd retired to Fort Myers. We also took her to lots of restaurants and tourist attractions. It was wonderful to see Ruth and Howdy having such a good time, I only wish it could've lasted longer. After a week's visit, Ruth went back home to Pittsburgh, and we returned to our normal routine again.

Christmas came and went without too much happening, and we entered the New Year of 1982 on a happy note.

On January 10th, we all went to Tampa for some sightseeing and dinner. On our return trip, Harry started to complain about chest pains. At first, the pains were minor, and we thought it was probably just indigestion. We stopped at a gas station for some pop for Harry, but the pains kept coming. I wanted to stop somewhere and get Harry some medical assistance, but he said no. He promised we could stop at Humana Hospital and he'd get a check-up, if he still had the pains when we got back to Dade City.

By the time we got to Dade City, Harry was in severe pain, so we went straight to the hospital. After much testing and consulting, the doctors confirmed he was having a heart attack. They put him in an ambulance and sent him to Tampa General Hospital. The next day, he had open-heart surgery. What a scary experience that was!

That evening, when we got back from the hospital, I called Harry's son in Michigan and he flew down the next day. Harry made a rapid recovery, so after a few days, his son went back home.

Howdy and I made the trip back and forth to Tampa for several more days. We managed to get lost on several occasions, but eventually, we'd figure it out, and be on our way again.

One day when we got to the hospital, Howdy and I somehow went to the wrong building. We didn't realize our mistake right away. So we got into the elevator and went up several flights thinking we were going to be on the floor Harry was on. What a surprise! We got on the elevator again and rode it down to the ground level. After looking around, we were a bit embarrassed, but we headed for the correct building, and finally were back on the right track again. By the time we reached Harry's room, Howdy and I were exhausted. It was more frightening being lost in the hospital building than weaving through the maze of heavy traffic on the long trip home.

When Harry was dismissed from the hospital, a friend of ours, Walter Schmidt, drove us to Tampa and back home again so we didn't have to worry about being lost again. We certainly had wonderful friends in Florida.

Harry continued improving, and by March, he decided that he was healthy enough to make the trip back north again. So, in early March, he packed up and drove back to Michigan.

Howdy and I spent the year from March 1982 to March 1983 in the kind of blissful retirement married couples dream about. Little did we know what the following months would bring - the beginning of a devastating series of events that would change our lives forever.

CHAPTER 4 – THE TERRIBLE BEGINNING

Now, I'll relate Howdy's story, and tell you about all the frustrations and heartaches of dealing with Alzheimer's. Throughout the following narrative there will be entries of doctor's evaluations of Howdy.

April 1983

Up until April 1983, we were living in blissful serenity, and I never dreamed of our future problems.

Howdy had been having a little trouble urinating, but we didn't think it was serious enough to warrant a doctor's visit. Most days Howdy didn't seem to be in much pain, but there were days when he was, and somehow, I knew - even though he didn't complain about it. Then one day there was blood in his urine. That really worried me, so I called our family doctor, Dr. Hughes, and he had us come to his office so he could examine Howdy.

Some of the Doctor Hughes' comments:

April 22, 1983:

Physical exam: Howard looks fine. He is a pleasant gentleman. Blood pressure is 168/90. He is overweight. He is kind of short, he shouldn't weigh anywhere close to 186 pounds. Head and neck examination was negative. Chest and heart sounds were normal. Abdomen was soft. We did a rectal examination, 3+enlarged prostate. The Hemostat showed that Howdy was very tender much more so than I would have expected. The Hemostat showed negative on the stool though. He has well healed pyonidal cyst scars.

Assessment: Hematuria (bloody urine).

Plan: We did a urine analysis. I gave him Bactrim DS one po b.i.d. for the next three weeks, I would like to see him back in two weeks time. I think that a cystoscopy (an examination of the bladder with a cystoscope) is going to be necessary even with only one episode.

That was when Howdy began showing signs of unusual behavior. The primary change in Howdy was his sudden rebelliousness, which I'm sure was a result of his frustration at not fully understanding what was happening to him. He was also having more and more problems with forgetfulness, and he seemed to become angry at the drop of a hat. Things were beginning to happen to him that none of us could understand, and I was feeling uneasy and apprehensive myself. By the time we went back to see Dr. Hughes, I had an ominous feeling about what the future might hold for us.

May 6, 1983:
History and physical: Doing fine. He did have some blood in his underwear. He is taking Bactrim for two weeks now, he has had no further symptoms. Plan: I think he should see a urologist for a cystoscopy.

Based on the doctor's suggestion we made an appointment with Dr. Garcia, an urologist in Dade City. After testing Howdy, the doctor decided there was a problem with Howdy's prostate. Dr. Garcia's assessment was that Howdy had Hematuria, and he'd have to undergo an operation on his prostate. The operation was scheduled at the Dade City Hospital, which was a relief for me because I was afraid we'd have to travel back and forth to Tampa.

May 12, 1983
Howdy's surgery was performed at the Dade City Hospital on May 12, 1983. After the operation was over, and Howdy was back in his room, Doctor Garcia told me the operation went well. He said Howdy would probably stay in the hospital for a couple days, and then we could go back home and return to living a normal life. He even said we could resume having normal marital relations if we chose to do so.

After Howdy came out of the anesthesia he told me he was on the fourth floor. But there were only three floors at that hospital. Was he only dreaming? I don't know, but he was certain he was on the fourth floor, and he was adamant about it. That was one of the first instances of Howdy not thinking clearly. Since he was on quite a bit of pain medication after his operation, I blamed the medicines for anything he did that I considered unusual.

For the entire time Howdy was in the hospital, I stayed right with him as much as I possibly could. Deep down in my heart I really felt no one could take care of Howdy as well as I could. Much later, after so many excellent caregivers provided Howdy with wonderful care, I certainly changed my mind. I discovered that the people who helped take care of Howdy were some of the most well trained and caring people I ever met.

May 14, 1983

A couple days after Howdy's operation I went in to visit him early in the morning, and I noticed a large number of blood clots in the drainage jar. When Doctor Garcia arrived I asked him, "Why all the clots?" Evidently he had no idea they were there, at least not that many. He went hurrying down the hall for a nurse. Then it dawned on me that there weren't supposed to be any clots. For years I've wondered about those clots, and what effect they had on Howdy's health problems. For a long time I wondered if any of the clots could've broken loose and floated around in his body, and later on caused damage.

Following the operation, after Howdy came home, he seemed to behave normally and we held normal conversations. Then, I began to see some noticeable changes in the way he was acting. He became angry much more often. If I brought up something about the operation, he'd go from being perfectly calm to being extremely agitated. Since Howdy was usually a calm man, I began to worry about his suddenly explosive temper outbursts. But, at least at that point in time, when he became upset, he'd quickly calm down again.

I remember one time in particular when he found something lying on our kitchen counter that he didn't think belonged there. He just picked it up and threw it across the room. The first time he did that, I was quite bewildered, as I couldn't understand what would possess him to do such a thing. But after it happened again, I knew his personality had changed and I began to wonder if I could expect those types of behaviors from him thereafter.

In addition to his increased level of agitation, he began swearing at every little thing. Prior to this, he generally had some good reason to use an expletive. Suddenly, it seemed as if his favorite words were damn, hell, and bitch. In some ways, his excessive cussing was comical because I was the one in the family who swore at the drop of a hat. It was a little like watching myself in a mirror, and I found myself being a little more selective in my choice of words. Eventually, I learned to accept that particular change in Howdy.

June 2, 1983

The first major incident in Howdy's deteriorating health occurred a few weeks later, on a beautiful June day. It was a peaceful evening, and I was cleaning up the dishes and loading the dishwasher after dinner. Howdy was out on our screened in porch (he loved that porch, and spent most of his time out there). Suddenly, I heard a terrible crash and the sound of flowerpots breaking. I rushed out and found Howdy lying on the floor. He was covered with plants and soil, and lying next to a chair and coffee table that had been knocked over. I had a difficult time getting him on his feet and into the house. My first thought was to call the rescue squad and get him to the hospital. His speech was a little garbled and he didn't look good to me, but he kept begging me not to put him in the hospital. The word "hospital" seemed to terrify him. I think his recent stay in the hospital, when he had his prostate operation, really scared him, so we spent the night at home. Thankfully, he had a fairly good night – I think he actually slept better than I did that night.

First thing the next morning, I got in touch with Doctor Hughes, and he told me to bring Howdy in as soon as I could. That turned out to be quite a struggle because Howdy was extremely disoriented and very unsteady on his feet. In addition to that, he weighed quite a bit more than I did, so it took all the strength I could muster to move him at all. We took it one step at a time, and I finally managed to get Howdy into the car, and we hurried off to the doctor's office. To this day, I don't know how I was able to get him into the car that morning.

When we pulled into the parking lot of the doctor's office, we had a hard time finding a parking place close enough to allow me to get Howdy from the car to the office easily. Again, we had quite a struggle, but somehow we made it.

When I told the nurses my husband had a stroke, I expected them to treat the situation as if it were an emergency. They were so nonchalant - I just couldn't believe it! They took three more patients before they finally got around to calling Howdy. I felt, under the circumstances, the nursing staff should have noticed we were having a terrible time, and should have acted more quickly. Just watching me handle Howdy should have alerted them to my desperation. As usual, I expected more concern than we received.

When the doctor finally examined Howdy, he said he'd had a slight stroke. I asked him if he thought the clots had something to do with it. He simply said "No." I was never convinced, however.

June 3, 1983:

History and physical: Howard was found lying on the front porch last evening. When his wife finally got him on his feet she noticed that his mouth was sagging on the left side. He has recently been discharged after having prostate surgery. He is taking Bactrim for urinary infection but really nothing else.

Physical exam: Shows indeed that his speech is difficult, he has sagging at left corner of his mouth to gross examination. More detailed neurological revealed he is alert and oriented. His pupils are reacting, he had no nystagmus. His sensation was intact facially, however, he did have sagging of the left corner of his mouth. His gag reflex was intact, normal shoulder shrug. His tongue protruded in midline. Cerebellum - he just had a lot of discoordination of the left arm, 4+ in right, 3+ in the left leg, 4+ in the right. Toe is up going on the left side.

Assessment: Obvious CVA (Cerebral Vascular Accident).

Plan: We would like to admit him to the hospital for further work up, but he just absolutely refused. Therefore, we will make arrangements for home physical therapy, home visiting nurse, and outpatient CAT scan.

The doctor felt very strongly that Howdy should be hospitalized, but Howdy flatly refused to go. To get Howdy to a hospital, we'd have had to forcibly take him - he was that terrified. Therefore, the doctor made arrangements for nurses to home-visit Howdy. He also said he'd set up an outpatient CAT scan for Howdy at a clinic in Lakeland.

The doctor also put Howdy on sleeping pills hoping we'd get more sleep. The only problem with the sleeping pills was he didn't always want to get up the morning after taking one of the pills. I was never sure if I could get Howdy out of bed and dressed, especially early in the morning if we had to go someplace. Sometimes, the pills really knocked Howdy out, and other times they had no effect on him.

A couple days later Dr. Hughes called to tell me he'd arranged for Howdy to have the CAT scan. He explained there were several things that could be wrong with Howdy, and the scan would tell us if he had any permanent damage to his brain. It'd also let us know if any of his arteries were blocked. If the CAT scan didn't show any irregularities, then we might be facing the possibility that Howdy could have Alzheimer's disease. I'd heard of Alzheimer's, but I really didn't know very much about it at the time.

Over the next several days, Howdy began exhibiting behavioral patterns I'd never seen in him before. The most apparent change was in his general attitude – he seemed very belligerent whenever he faced a situation he didn't understand. He seemed especially resentful of anyone who tried to exert authority over him. Within a week of the stroke, Howdy was physically back to normal. But his behavior patterns were anything but normal. Another major change in his behavior was when Howdy began showing signs of restlessness – but not all the time. On some days, he seemed to be constantly on the move, walking from room to room, sitting down for few minutes, then up again and roaming about, then down, and up again. The next day, he'd be perfectly normal in every way. On the days he was so restless, I noticed he'd suddenly focus his eyes on an object, but it was as if he didn't know what the object was, or how to use it. Sometimes I'd try to explain something to him, but he didn't seem to understand what I was trying to tell him. Then I'd have to talk to him like he was a child, and explain everything in great detail.

CHAPTER 5 – LAKELAND CLINIC

On the morning of Howdy's appointment in Lakeland, we walked into the Clinic, and it looked as if half of the senior citizens in that part of Florida were crowded into the waiting room. If you've ever been to a clinic you know how much time you spend just waiting. As luck would have it, that happened to be one of Howdy's bad days, and being with someone who had no idea why he had to sit and wait made the waiting extremely stressful for me. He wouldn't sit still for more than a few minutes, so we were constantly up and down. None of the doctor's staff got excited, or even seemed to rush at all to get us in quickly.

Eventually, after a preliminary examination, and more waiting, it was time for the CAT scan. We had to go to another department on another floor. We also sat there for a long time, and Howdy became even more restless. When they finally called his name, I got up to take Howdy in. When the nurse told me I couldn't go with him, I laughed to myself. She just didn't understand how hard he was to handle. I tried to explain that to the nurse, but she didn't want to listen to me. I was especially concerned because there was no way of knowing when something would catch Howdy's eye, and he'd grab it and either hurt himself, or possibly break it. I tried again to convince the nurse that I really needed to be with Howdy, because she was not going to be able to handle him. She told me they were trained for all kinds of emergencies. I knew she was in for a surprise, but I decided to let her find out for herself.

I waited as she headed down the long hallway with Howdy in tow. I could see Howdy was struggling to break loose. Then, suddenly, I heard someone calling out in a loud, panicky voice, "**Mrs. Weidman! Come here, Mrs Weidman – Please, hurry!**" (I hate to admit it, but I did get some satisfaction out of that, although I resisted the temptation to say, "I told you so."). I rushed to catch up with them, and I could see she really was having a hard time with Howdy.

When we got to the CAT scan room, I insisted on holding Howdy's hand and helping him onto the table as I explained what they needed him to do.

It took quite a bit of coaxing to get him on the examining table. Why he had to be put on a table, and into a machine that looked like a very confining cylinder, was simply too much for him to comprehend. After he settled down, I couldn't move too far away, because it really upset him if I wasn't in sight. I had to stay with him for the entire procedure. As long as I was right there, he was cooperative. It took a lot of sweet talk, but the scanner finally clicked off, and then he was all right. The nurses were very polite, and thanked me for helping them with Howdy (it seemed the deeper we got into Alzheimer's, the more dependent Howdy was on me - he wanted me in his sight constantly).

After making it through the CAT scan ordeal, we waited again to see the neurologist. It seemed like another interminable wait, but finally, we were taken into his office and I helped Howdy into a seat. I took an instant dislike to the neurologist. I got the impression he didn't have much experience with people who were exhibiting the unusual types of behaviors I'd observed in Howdy. And if he didn't have experience with these cases before, I doubted that he could understand what we were going through. Even so, I could've respected his opinion if he had been sympathetic and caring, but he wasn't at all. He really never seemed to talk to me seriously about Howdy's condition. Most of Howdy's doctors were at least willing to take the time to discuss things with me, and ask me questions about what I'd observed, but I never got that feeling with the neurologist.

During Howdy's neurological evaluation, the neurologist was very short with me. I had the feeling he not only didn't understand what I was going through with Howdy, but he didn't care, either. He probably thought his cool approach was the best way to handle a potentially hysterical woman, but I was having a great deal of difficulty trying to cope with Howdy's strange behaviors, and I needed consoling and understanding. Later on, once we moved back to Ohio, our doctor up there understood my emotional state far better, and I felt he handled me in the right way. Consequently, he and I got along very well.

Many of the doctors and nurses we dealt with wouldn't listen to me when I tried to tell them about the things Howdy did. I know they each had a medical education I didn't have, but I lived with Howdy and his condition. When I explained to the doctors about the bizarre things Howdy did, they'd have a look of disbelief on their faces. Some of the things he did, I never told anyone. I just couldn't. Someday, maybe I'll be able to tell everything. But until then, much of what transpired will remain a secret. The things written here, I feel at ease with. But a lot of secrets will be just between Howdy and me.

On the 16th of June 1983, Howdy's brother William (Howdy was the oldest son in a family of six children) passed away in Pennsylvania. We wanted to make the trip, but when I called the doctor, he advised against travel. I realized I had to make a difficult decision, and that Howdy's family might not understand, but we just couldn't go.

Thereafter, we went through a period where Howdy simply didn't want to do almost anything I told him to do, and he also began exhibiting more bizarre behaviors. We were both learning to cope with circumstances as they were, however. I had to learn to coax and persuade him into doing some of the things he didn't want to do. For example, if I told him to change his shoes, he might take off the pair he had on, but then he'd refuse to put on the other pair. So I'd try to convince him he really wanted to put the shoes on. Sometimes, I had to tell him several times before he'd respond. I couldn't always use the same tactics, as he didn't respond in the same way each time. On some occasions, I even had to have him take his socks off and start from scratch, so ultimately, he'd put his shoes on.

About that same time, Howdy was having an increasingly harder time trying to remember how to do things. A simple thing like getting into the shower stall became a big problem. He couldn't seem to figure out which foot went in first. Even when he got the first foot in, that wasn't the end of the problem, because there were times when he didn't know what to do next.

Although Howdy would occasionally act completely out of character, he still managed to function normally most of the time. That was one of the things about Alzheimer's I had a hard time understanding. How could Howdy be so out of it one minute, and the very next minute go back to being his old self again? On his better days, of which there were still quite a few, we were still able to enjoy being with our friends and Herbert and Sylvia. Sylvia was a very good cook, and we enjoyed lots of delicious, home-cooked meals at their house.

In Florida, there was always something to do, or some really neat places to visit. We all enjoyed going to different restaurants for meals, which, of course, meant none of us had to cook when we went on one of our excursions. Most of the restaurants we visited were beautifully landscaped, and all of them had fancy gift shops that carried lots of interesting souvenirs. We spent many happy hours just looking at the wide variety of items that each gift shop offered for sale.

Howdy actually took to those little excursions quite well. He was always well behaved when we went into a restaurant, or gift shop, and he'd tell me how nice some of the items were. I was so glad he was always very careful when he handled the souvenirs. Even our friends commented on his keen awareness of his surroundings.

I never had to worry about what to do when Howdy needed to use the restroom, because one of the men in our crowd would escort Howdy and take good care of him while he was in there. I was relieved that the men never treated Howdy differently. They all made a point of including Howdy in every conversation, and he seemed to respond to the attention quite well. I thought he really liked hearing different voices, instead of just hearing my voice all the time.

I also remember how delighted he'd be when I told him we were going touring some place, and other people would be going with us. Howdy liked getting all dressed up and I'd always ask him what he wanted to wear. I tried to let him make most of his decisions himself. I thought it was important for him to feel as if he were still in control of some aspects of his life.

He'd seem genuinely excited when we headed into the bedroom to pick out what he'd be wearing for the day. Most of the time, he picked out a nice pair of pants, a matching shirt, a nice sweater, and last, but not least, his navy blue cowboy hat.

Throughout the remainder of 1983, we made several more visits to Doctor Hughes in Dade City, and he continued trying different medicines in an attempt to help Howdy. I don't think he was sure how to attack the problem, because I was convinced Alzheimer's was still a relatively unknown disease to the medical profession in the early eighties. It seemed no matter what the doctor tried, he was still guessing. One of the drugs Doctor Hughes prescribed was Haldol. Howdy took Haldol for some time, and the best I can say is that it may have slowed the deterioration of his condition, but unfortunately, it didn't reverse the symptoms.

CHAPTER 6 – AN ENDLESS NIGHTMARE

January 24, 1984:

History and physical: Howard has been dizzy for the last 24 hours. It came on suddenly and actually described true vertigo quite nicely. It is associated with some nausea and he has vomited.

Physical exam: Shows that he looks fine today. He has no rotary or horizontal nystagmus. His fundoscopic was negative. He had no cartoid bruits or palpable thyroid. Heart sounds were normal. No murmurs on systoli or diastoli. Chest was otherwise clear.

Assessment: Acute labyrinthitis, viral.

Plan: Antivert 12.5 one po t.i.d., if he is not improved he will return.

Some of our doctor visits were uneventful. Nothing of consequence came from most of the visits, such as the one above when Howdy had a virus.

Throughout the year 1984 Howdy went from acting and conversing normally to bizarre behaviors and incoherent speech about fifty percent of the time. One day he'd be as normal as ever and we'd talk as we always did, then the next day, he'd be "off in space" somewhere. And it wasn't always a day to day change. The change in Howdy could take place at just about any time of the day or night. He might get up one day, and be perfectly normal in every way. I might leave him in the house long enough to mow the grass, and by the time I came back in, he'd have a glazed look in his eyes and I knew he was "off" again. Whenever he had that lost look on his face I never knew what to expect from him. Even though he seemed to be agitated at times when he was "out of it," a great deal of the time he'd be smiling. When his anger was under control, he seemed to think everything that happened was funny.

Sometimes, even on one of his "off" days, if I took the time to really listen to what he was saying, his conversations would be very intelligent sounding. I tried so hard to engage him in conversation during those times, even if we only discussed the weather – anything, just to keep him talking became very important to me.

When Howdy looked exceptionally lost or forlorn, I'd stand in front of him and hug him. Then I'd look him in the eye, and ask him, "Where did Howdy go?" He'd get very serious, and look at me and say, "I just don't know." He seemed as perplexed as I was.

The next phase in Howdy's behavior swings included roaming aimlessly all over the house, and even outside. He seemed to be constantly on the go, and along with his increased level of activity, he seemed to be in a constant state of agitation. I could never relax completely, because I never knew what he might get into next. It was like he was constantly looking for something. I never understood what he was looking for, nor do I believe he knew, but night and day he was continually on the move. I had the impression he really didn't know where he was, and not understanding what he was doing in such a strange place must have been terribly frightening to him.

He also seemed to be constantly worried about the time of day. Time was very important to him. He was always looking at the clock. He insisted the grandfather clock needed winding, and he wanted to pull the chains. When I told him, "no!" he got very upset. We went through a period where he was always moving, walking around, trying to outwit me to get to the clock. It was just a matter of who outlasted whom. He also wanted to compare the grandfather clock to his wristwatch all the time, and if there were just a few minutes difference he'd ask me why. Naturally, I never had the right answer. There were even times when I'd catch him looking at his watch and counting off the minutes as each one passed.

Some nights he'd sleep for only a few minutes at a time - if he slept for an hour and a half I considered it a bonus. It never occurred to me the day would come when he'd sleep so long I'd be alarmed. Later on, I lost count of how many trips I made to the bedroom to make sure he was still breathing. It was odd, but when he didn't sleep, I worried, and when he did sleep, I still worried. There simply wasn't a time when I didn't worry about him.

Howdy came up with a new wrinkle for me when he got the notion the furniture needed moved. He spent the next several weeks moving furniture from one place to another. I'd find kitchen chairs in the living room, dining room chairs out on the front porch, and porch furniture in the living room, or dining room. When he tried to move the heavy china closet, I really began to worry. If I hadn't stopped him, what would have happened? If he'd have knocked that over, every piece of good china we owned would have been destroyed. Also, if it had fallen on top of him, it might have killed him. I finally convinced myself it was better to have our china in pieces than to have a husband who was all banged up.

I love knick-knacks, and over the years, we managed to collect quite a few. The knick-knacks never seemed to be where Howdy thought they should be. So he moved them, again, and again, and again. He'd also empty out all the drawers, over and over. For some reason, he didn't bother with the lamps. After moving everything, he'd turn around and put everything back in its rightful place. I was exhausted just watching him. But, as long as he wasn't hurting himself, or the furniture, it was easier to just let him do his thing than to try to stop him. When he began moving the glasses around, it scared me a little bit. I didn't want him getting cut, but he was really very careful. I was constantly amazed at just how gentle Howdy was in handling breakables.

One day he asked me for a cloth. After I gave him one, he went into the living room and dusted all the furniture. For some reason he never asked to push the sweeper. I think the noise of the motor bothered him.

On another day, I needed some hot water to rinse out some things. But when I turned on the faucets, the water was cold. I looked at all the faucets around the house, but they were all off (Howdy loved to turn on the faucets). So, I decided to wait an hour and try again, but still no hot water. After several hours, it finally occurred to me to go out to the utility sink in the shed. Sure enough, both of the faucets were on full blast. I still don't know how Howdy managed to slip by me to get to the shed that day. Because Howdy moved so slowly most of the time, I was surprised at how fast he could move when he really wanted to.

During that year, there were many mysteries I was unable to solve. In the beginning, I'd get so frustrated and angry I'd yell at Howdy, but that only made matters worse. My anger would upset him very much. I soon discovered the most important thing for me was to get my own emotions under control, because if I didn't, it might send Howdy over the edge. On those occasions when I did have an outburst, I felt such terrible remorse I just wanted to beg Howdy to forgive me. The aching in my heart, and my anger at myself for being such a fool, were never ending. The "I'm so sorry's," would start all over again. Then I'd hold Howdy in my arms, and tenderly tell him how much I loved him. Sometimes, I felt so terrible I wanted to die. I desperately wanted to make up for all the hurt I'd caused him - but I couldn't undo what I'd done.

I knew something had to change. I didn't want to turn into a screamer, or a hysterical woman. I had to sort things out and figure out how I could help Howdy without going insane myself, and to do that I'd need some help from God. I learned to pray a lot more often than I ever had before, and in the long run, my prayers were answered. The days ahead would be very trying, but I began to handle things much better.

Thus began the remaking of me. After yelling at Howdy one day, and watching the painful look that came over his face, I finally came to the realization I had to change. And boy did I! It took some time, but the change in my temperament really paid off in the end. I worked hard at it, and consequently I improved at caring for Howdy. And if I could've looked into a crystal ball, I'd have seen things were going to be completely different during the last five years, beginning in 1988. I wasn't the same person at all. Howdy could've done anything, and it wouldn't have bothered me. In fact, I learned the most valuable lesson of all, to laugh when our many disasters occurred. When something terrible happened, I'd wrap my arms around him, and whisper in his ear, "It's okay Howdy, we'll take care of it." I must have said those words a thousand of times. Somehow, I think he knew what I was telling him.

One of my habits at that time was to bring in the mail, and if I happened to be busy, I'd put it down until I had a free moment to read it later. You'd have thought, sooner or later, I'd figure out that wasn't the smartest thing to do, because every once in a while, I couldn't find the mail when I went to read it. Howdy evidently didn't think mail should be lying around, so he'd hide it, or throw it in the trash. When I realized my mistake, the hunt would be on again - once he even put the mail back in the mailbox.

Howdy didn't seem to like the idea of trash collecting in a trash container, either. It never surprised me to find one of the bathroom rubbish cans dumped in the sink, commode, on the floor, or in the tub. One day, I found a whole box of Q-tips in the commode.

From time to time, I'd send an audio tape to my son and his family in Ohio. When I'd mention some of the incidents on the tape, Howdy would listen and laugh - he thought it was quite funny. I guess he didn't realize I was talking about him. He truly seemed to enjoy listening to me tell those stories. He even tried to talk into the microphone every once in a while.

Another afternoon, when Harry was with us during his annual visit, we'd just finished lunch, and Harry and I were starting to get up from the table. Suddenly, Harry stopped me, "Look at Howdy!" Harry exclaimed. I looked at Howdy in time to see him spread jelly on his paper napkin, and then start to eat it. I asked him, "Wouldn't you rather have the jelly on some bread", and he answered, "Of course I would." So I made him a sandwich on bread, and that seemed to be much more to his liking. Despite that incident, and many others, Harry refused to believe Howdy was really ill. For several years, even as Howdy became progressively worse, Harry stubbornly insisted Howdy was only faking his condition to gain attention. As time went on, his unrelenting attitude drove a wedge between us, and I felt differently about Harry.

Howdy liked to go riding in the car, so I took him for a drive as often as I could. He never seemed to care where we went. He just wanted to go. One day, we went to Hardee's for some hamburgers, and then we took them home to eat. I put Howdy on a chair in the living room with a TV table and his hamburger. I got busy, and a few minutes later, when I looked at him, I noticed he wasn't eating anymore. I knew there hadn't been enough time for him to finish his hamburger, but I couldn't find it anywhere. A couple minutes later he tried to stand up, but he fell back into his chair and began moaning. Something was obviously bothering him. He tried to stand again, and once again fell back into the chair. After he tried to get up the third time, I decided to ask him what was wrong. He told me his foot was hurting, so I took off his right shoe, and there was the hamburger crammed into the toe of the shoe. It seemed as if the impossible tasks came easy for him. After I disposed of the mangled hamburger and put his shoe back on, I asked him if he was still hungry. He said he was, so I made him another lunch.

Another day, I prepared Howdy a nice, big lunch. He ate every bit of it, but ten minutes later he said, "Aren't we going to have any lunch today?" So I went back to the kitchen, made him another complete lunch, and he ate every bite. Even though he was full, his brain told him he was still hungry.

When Howdy was still able to dress himself, we had some very amusing incidents. Quite often, his shoes would end up on the wrong feet. Sometimes, he'd put his shoes on, and then he'd try to put his socks on over his shoes. I couldn't help but laugh, and when he'd see me laughing, he'd start laughing, too. Occasionally, I'd ask him if he was trying to keep his shoes warm, and then he'd start to laugh again. He'd say, "Boy, are they ever cold!"

Howdy was still able to play shuffleboard that year and I think he really enjoyed the companionship of our friends and neighbors. Unfortunately, our shuffleboard days were also drawing to a close, as we were about to enter into a new phase of Howdy's illness.

CHAPTER 7 – SEIZURES AND MORE BIZARRE BEHAVIORS

In March of 1985, Howdy and I were taking a walk around the park when he suddenly stumbled and almost fell over. If I hadn't been close enough to grab him, he might've taken a bad fall. Just before he stumbled, I felt him trembling so violently I almost thought I was the one trembling. He didn't seem to have any other symptoms, so I let him gather himself for a few moments, and then we continued on our walk. I kind of panicked momentarily when I thought he had a seizure of some sort. But when he snapped out of it right away, I thought maybe I was overreacting. I decided it was better not to alarm him by letting him see how concerned I was, so I tried to act nonchalant. What I didn't realize at the time was that he'd have more episodes like this one over the next couple of years. Even though there were not a great number of seizures, that first one really startled me. At that point, I realized another change had taken place in Howdy. So, I decided Howdy needed to see Dr. Hughes again.

March 18, 1985:

History and physical: Yesterday Howdy almost fell over, his wife grabbed him. He didn't actually fall down, he had no seizure activity, and he had no warning. He is susceptible to CVA's, etc. He did have one syncopal episode about 3 months ago. He looks fine, bright, and alert. BP is 150/80, pulse is regular for 2 min., no carotid bruits, pupils reactive, fundoscopic neg., neurologically; he's intact.

Assessment: Presyncope.

Plan: We'll get an EEG, 24 hr. Holtor monitor, he's had a CAT scan, I'll notify him of the results and I'll see him in a week.

Although Doctor Hughes did not think Howdy had a seizure, I wasn't convinced (after Howdy had additional episodes, we agreed he had, indeed, had a series of seizures).

Dr. Hughes set up an appointment for us at the Humana Hospital in Dade City for an EEG the next day. Even something as simple as an EEG, however, was frightening to Howdy. When the doctor told me I'd have to take Howdy to the hospital for the procedure, I had to do some real fast talking to convince Howdy to go. After I explained everything in great detail, Howdy said, "Okay." I was quite relieved when the visit came off without incident.

Our follow-up visit to Dr. Hughes confirmed what I'd been thinking.

March 26 1985:

History and physical: He's getting along pretty well, He's occasionally belligerent now, which is typical of OBS. His EEG was abnormal, and the spells he's having could well be mild seizure activity. Try Dilantin.

Plan: we'll 100 mg t.i.d. x 3 months, I'll see him back, If belligerence continues, we'll start him on Haldol, he's had a normal CAT scan in 1983.

A few months later, he had a second episode, which was similar to the first with trembling and shaking. Once again, if I hadn't had a good grip on him he surely would have fallen.

Throughout 1985 our trips to the doctor's office became more frequent because of Howdy's seizures. It seemed as if the seizures also triggered changes in Howdy's behavior. One change was that he had even more angry outbursts than he'd had before. Even though Doctor Hughes could find no reason for the seizures, and consequently, for his changes in behavior, I felt he should examine Howdy whenever he had an episode. Thankfully, Howdy had only a few more episodes during 1985.

After the first two seizures, none of the others happened during the daylight hours - they always occurred at night. I'd be sleeping soundly, only to be awakened by a terrible shaking of the bed. Then I'd find Howdy shaking violently, but he never cried out, or made any sounds at all. The seizures lasted for only a few minutes, not long enough for me to summon the rescue squad. After a few minutes of trembling, Howdy would return to being normal again. He never had any type of damage the doctor could detect after an episode, so the doctor was never able to determine what caused the seizures.

When Howdy did have a seizure, it scared me half to death. Even though it was just a brief period of time, he'd be so terribly convulsed I had no idea what to do to help him. It was a frightfully helpless feeling watching someone in that state, and to be powerless to do anything about it.

After the episode in March, Howdy began to say nasty things to me from time to time. Through all the years Howdy and I were married, we never really had any arguments, and he was very easy to get along with. I knew other women whose husbands were verbally abusive, but I can honestly say Howdy never talked to me like that. You can imagine my surprise one-day when I asked him how he was, and he looked me square in the eye and said very plainly "Go to hell!" To say I was surprised would be a major understatement. Shocked would be a much better way to describe my reaction. After that day, he'd give me a smart answer every once in a while. Thankfully, he didn't talk to me like that on a daily basis.

May 29,1985:

History and physical: He's doing well, his short-term memory is shot, he doesn't know my name, or the day, but otherwise he's doing fine. He's a little verbally abusive with his wife, but not serious. They're getting ready to go on a three-month trip, which is worrisome.

I'd told Dr. Hughes we were planning to visit our family in Ohio for about three months, but after thinking it over, I decided Howdy wouldn't do well for that length of time away from home. We ended up spending most of that summer in Florida because I never knew when Howdy would have a mood change, and I didn't want the family to see him like that.

I finally decided we'd spend the month of July in Ohio and Pennsylvania. That would give us enough time to see our son, his wife, and our grandchildren, and still have time to visit Howdy's family in Pittsburgh, and also visit my sister and her family in Aliquippa.

When I talked to Howdy about going to Ohio and Pennsylvania, he seemed quite pleased and he told me he was looking forward to the trip. Since July was a very hot month in Florida, I figured it couldn't be any hotter up north.

We had a nice trip to Ohio, and Howdy did seem to enjoy the drive because he liked riding in the car. Since Howdy couldn't do any of the driving, it was up to me to do it all. I was in pretty good health, and I really enjoyed driving, so it turned out to be a happy trip for both of us.

To make the trip less tiresome, I decided we should stop and visit our niece, Bonnie Bever and her family in South Carolina. We truly enjoyed our time with them. Bonnie always took us shopping at the outlet malls in South Carolina whenever we visited. Even though we didn't spend much money, Howdy and I got a big kick out of going to the malls.

The Bevers lived in a very nice, new mobile home, and the view from the back of their house was spectacular. They were so close to the mountains that it seemed as if you could reach out and touch them. One day, they took us up one of the mountains, and I have to confess I have a fear of heights, so it turned out to be a scary trip for me. Howdy, on the other hand, loved that trip, and I was glad we went up that mountain for his sake. The view from up there was wonderful. We had such a nice time we hated to leave.

The trip to South Carolina had taken about ten hours, and we were looking at another ten-hour trip from there to Delaware, Ohio. Because I love to drive so much, it seemed like a much shorter trip. Howdy not only enjoyed the drive, but he also loved to listen to music, and we were well supplied with lots of audio tapes. So, we cruised along listening to music tapes as well as listening to the radio. Since I'm not a lover of the newer music, I enjoyed listening to the old-time singers. Howdy and I both liked to sing, or hum, to the music, which made the trip much more pleasant. If names like Jim Nabors, Johnny Mathis, or Nat "King" Cole, and the big band hits of the 30s and 40s sound familiar, that's the kind of music we listened to on our trips.

Finally, we arrived in Delaware early in July. What a welcome sight that was after such a long journey. When you haven't seen your family for about a year, it's really nice to see them again. Throughout our trip, Howdy was on his best behavior, and we were able to spend pleasant times with our family that summer. We also were able to see most of Howdy's family in Pittsburgh, and Mary Jane and her family in Aliquippa. I felt we were fortunate to see just about everyone we wanted to see, because I wasn't sure what Howdy would be like the next time those folks saw him. Howdy especially seemed to enjoy seeing his two sisters, Ruth and Grace, who lived together in Pittsburgh.

On the trip back home, we again stayed with Bonnie and her family for a couple days in South Carolina. We had a nice visit, but by then, Howdy and I were pretty eager to get home.

I had to laugh as we neared Dade City because Howdy told me where to make the turns. The closer we got to home, the more landmarks he recognized. The ups and downs of Alzheimer's never ceased to amaze me. When Howdy told me to turn into the park, he had the biggest grin on his face that I ever saw. Then, out of the blue, he yelled, "We're home!" He truly did love Florida. I really enjoyed that summer, and I think Howdy had a good time as well. At least he smiled a lot, and most of the time he was able to talk normally with everyone. All in all, we had a wonderful trip.

At that time, we were only going back to Ohio for short periods of time, and since we didn't have our own place up there, we always stayed with family. Now I think back on it, I really think it was hard on them. But no one ever complained, and they always welcomed us with open arms and always asked us to stay longer.

Once we returned home after our trip north, Howdy began falling out of bed, (sometimes three or four times a night). We weren't getting much sleep to begin with, but when he started falling out of bed, we got a lot less sleep. Once he was on the floor, it was a major project getting him back in bed, and by the time I did, I was always wide-awake. Because he didn't know his right from his left, up from down, arms from legs, etc. it was virtually impossible to give him directions as he had no idea what I was talking about. I quickly learned I had to talk to him in a very soft voice, repeat what I was telling him over and over, and finally we'd get it done. I used tactile cues as much as possible such as patting the leg or arm I wanted him to move, and in time, I got through to him and we'd get him back in bed.

Shortly after we returned to Florida following our summer vacation, we scheduled an appointment with Dr. Hughes. Unfortunately, due to Howdy's increased inactivity, and all the wonderful food we were treated to, he was gradually getting heavier. His condition was also getting progressively worse. He couldn't seem to remember anything. Even something simple that had been a part of his daily routine for his entire adult life, like shaving, was now pretty much beyond his comprehension.

CHAPTER 8 – COGENTIN

I remember the year 1985 as the most trying year of all. It seemed to be for a number of reasons. First of all, some of the things Howdy did, such as putting his shoes on the wrong feet, or urinating in the bathtub were becoming more commonplace. He seemed even more unable to figure out how to do some of the simplest tasks that he needed to do, like bringing his chair closer to the table. Or he'd keep trying to put his false teeth in his mouth upside down, and then not be able to figure out why it didn't work that way.

On the other hand, there were also several repetitive behaviors that seemed to occupy his mind for extended periods of time. For example, he went through a period where he continually counted his fingers, and every once in a while, he'd do it correctly. When he didn't, I'd tell him to try again, and quite often, on the second or third try, he'd, finally, get it right. But on those occasions when he just couldn't seem to figure it out, frustration would take over. At those times, he became extremely hard to control.

Howdy liked ketchup on his omelets, but sometimes he'd put ketchup on his toast instead of his eggs. One morning at breakfast, he kept putting heaping spoonfuls of sugar in his coffee. Before I could stop him, he put at least six spoonfuls in his cup. I couldn't leave the salt shaker on the table either, because he'd use it profusely - he simply didn't know when to stop.

On another occasion, he asked me for a pair of socks. I thought for some reason he wanted to change his socks, so I handed him a pair. I was quite busy at that moment, so I didn't pay much attention to what he was doing. When I finally looked at him, he had the socks on his hands. He managed to pull them all the way up to his elbows, and he was still trying to pull them up higher when I stopped him.

When Howdy disappeared into the back of the house for any length of time, on a day when I forgot to lock the door, he usually came out with a big grin on his face. I just knew he did something he thought was wonderful.

What he considered wonderful usually turned out to be a disaster for me. One day, when he did that, I asked him why he had a big grin. He wouldn't tell me, but he just kept smiling. So, I took him back to the bedroom, where I discovered all of the contents of the dresser drawers had been emptied onto the bed. As disasters went, that one wasn't too bad, except I couldn't find everything. It seemed like I couldn't take my eyes off of him for a second that entire year.

August 16, 1985:

History and physical: His OBS is just progressively worse. He is becoming a little combative now. His short-term memory is almost completely gone. His ability to perform normal daily tasks is becoming less and less, example he has great difficulty shaving.

Physical Exam: Shows he is confused. He absolutely has no short-term memory what so ever. Not oriented to time, place, or person. Otherwise, he looks physically fine. He has gained a lot of weight.

Assessment: OBS, probably Alzheimer's

Plan: I have increased his 30 at Haldol to 2 mg. b.i.d.,added Cogentin 2 mg. B.i.d. to his regimen. Some Restoril 30 at hs. He is up most of the night. Return in two weeks.

Howdy took Haldol for over two years, and while taking it his condition slowly deteriorated. It didn't seem to make Howdy particularly worse, but it didn't seem to make him any better, either. Therefore, Doctor Hughes made what was, in retrospect, a terrible decision - he prescribed Cogentin for Howdy. Since he hadn't had much experience treating patients who were suffering from Alzheimer's, I'm sure the radical changes in Howdy's behavior, as a result of his taking Cogentin, were just as surprising to Dr. Hughes as they were to me.

The doctor told me to give the new medication to Howdy for two weeks, and get back to him. My biggest mistake was not calling him after the second pill. Those pills turned Howdy into an absolute maniac! It's difficult to describe what a terrible change took place in Howdy's personality. How I lasted a week with him in that state, I'll never know. But I waited for an entire week before I called the doctor again.

Things happened in the week Howdy took Cogentin, and for many months thereafter, that weren't supposed to happen to patients with Alzheimer's for several years after the onset of the disease. During the fateful week Howdy was on that damnable drug, it was like all hell broke loose. Howdy had always been a mild mannered man, so when his behavior changed so drastically, it was a shock. He did things like chase me around the kitchen counter with a butcher knife. He angrily slammed the car door into the carport pole, threw plants out onto the walk, swore more than I ever heard him swear, and used the F-word, which I'd never heard him use before. Normal, everyday happenings would throw him into an uncontrollable rage.

During that week, it seemed whatever I told him to do, he was determined to defy me. If I told him it was time to eat, he acted as if he wasn't hungry - even if he really was. When he thought I didn't care, he'd suddenly become hungry. I also had to be sure I didn't leave the hoses lying around in the yard, because he'd turn the water on and spray the house. That wouldn't have been such a bad thing, except we lived in Florida, so we had the windows open night and day. After his watering episodes, I had to go around the house and wipe up all of the water that had soaked everything near a window. You'd have thought all the terrible things he did would've made me so watchful that, in time, I would've been a step ahead of him. But it was amazing how many times he managed to get ahead of me.

One day during that week, while Howdy was napping, I decided to mow the neighbor's yard. Suddenly, I thought I heard water running, so I hurried home. There was Howdy washing the car with the car windows wide open! In time, my hearing became so attuned to the sound of running water that, even if I was in the yard next door, that sound threw me into a panic. After one of those incidents, I was sure I heard Howdy saying, "She won't let me do anything!" Later, during that week of Howdy's most bizarre behaviors, I discovered he'd put several knives in the disposal. Luckily, I noticed the handles sticking out before I turned it on.

Another change occurred when Howdy didn't want to take a shower. He'd always been so good about personal cleanliness that that behavioral change was particularly surprising. At least that aversion to taking a shower lasted only a couple of weeks. It continually amazed me how quickly he'd go in and out of those little quirks. Some days he'd go into the shower stall willingly, then on the next day, I'd have to coax him and talk to him in a very soft voice to convince him it was all right. If that seemed to be working, I'd very gently inch him into the stall and the rest would be easy.

After a week of those terrible happenings, I finally called Dr. Hughes. When I told him how Howdy was reacting to the Cogentin, he told me to stop giving it to Howdy. Was I ever glad to hear that! When I tried to tell him I thought he'd given Howdy the wrong medicine, he said, "No way! Howdy's just had a bad reaction to the Cogentin." He could afford to be cavalier about it, but I had to live with what it did to Howdy – Doctor Hughes didn't. Later on, he admitted he had another patient who had the same reaction to Cogentin that Howdy did. I grew up in an era when people held all doctors in very high esteem, so I tried to follow the doctor's orders, even if my good judgement told me otherwise. Now, I know better.

The dramatic change in Howdy's demeanor had a profound effect on me as well. The situation was made worse by the fact neither Howdy, nor I, got much sleep, and not getting enough sleep was beginning to tell on me. For several days and nights at a time, Howdy didn't seem to need much sleep. Then, all of a sudden, for a day or two, he'd sleep pretty well. Overall, we had quite a few more sleepless nights than we had restful ones. No wonder I was so irritable.

When we went back to Dr. Hughes for our next visit, I wasn't sure who the doctor needed to treat more urgently – Howdy, or me.

August 30, 1985:
History and physical: He's getting worse, his wife can barely take care of him. He seems to have slipped a lot. The Cogentin and Haldol didn't help a bit.
Plan: I've made arrangements for immediate neurological evaluation.

That was the most frightening time for us. I'll never forget it. The doctor had no idea what it was like to go through those terrible days and nights. Between not getting enough sleep, and Howdy's bizarre behaviors, I was sure I was going through personality changes myself. Howdy wasn't the only one who was upset - I was, too. That was when Dr. Hughes said he started to see a difference in me, and I suppose, that's why he decided to evaluate me.

During our visit to Doctor Hughes, after the episode with the Cogentin, he asked me a lot of questions about my feelings. By that time, I was almost out of my mind. The doctor wrote in his evaluation, "Mrs. Weidman is having a great deal of difficulty coping with Howdy's behavioral abnormalities." If ever there was an understatement - that was it! There were days when I was continually on the verge of hysteria. One day, I called the neurologist because I was sobbing uncontrollably. He got really mad at me, and told me to, "Get hold of yourself and take care of your husband." He had no idea what good care I was giving Howdy. How could he, when he only saw us briefly on the day Howdy had his CAT scan? Fortunately, I finally got myself together for the long road ahead.

Even though Howdy only took the Cogentin for one week, it was as if his condition deteriorated much more rapidly thereafter. And there were many more instances of Howdy exhibiting bizarre behavior patterns from that time forward. For example, Howdy would take all of the silverware out of the drawers and place each one, piece by piece, in every part of the house.

And it wasn't unusual to find a pair of sox inside a glass in the cupboard, or in a cup. Once I found his under shorts in the freezer, and another time, I found them in the dishwasher. I never knew what I'd find in the dishwasher, the oven, a closet, or out on the porch. Every time Howdy passed the stove he'd touch the burners (I guess he was trying to see if they were on or off). I constantly had the worry about what would happen if I left them on. I had to be watchful all the time. I tried not to make any mistakes. And I always had the nagging worry of whether or not I was doing the right thing.

Periodically, I'd go to the back of the house only to find all of the sheets, pillowcases, and towels laid out over every open space he could find. Whenever I'd discover his handiwork, everything was folded neatly and in small stacks. For some reason he had a lot of patience doing those kinds of things. He could sit and fold and unfold his handkerchief for hours.

During that time, we tried all kinds of things to occupy his mind and keep him busy. His favorite activity was a child's plastic, stacking toy that entertained him for hours on end. It was a spindle with four or five different colored rings to be fitted on the spindle. That toy continued to amuse him for years. It was one of the best investments I ever made for him, and only a couple dollars.

Howdy loved to dress and undress. It wasn't unusual for him to come out of the bedroom with two or three pairs of pants on. They'd all be zippered, belted and the legs were all down to his shoe tops. Shirts would be the same way. They'd be buttoned and tucked in, and collars flat. He didn't just do these things once in a while, but over and over again. Finally, I had so much trouble keeping up with him I decided to put a lock on the bedroom door, not to lock him in, but to keep him out during the day. I felt, if he were confined to less space, I could keep up with him better. That kept him limited to the front of the house. It was also one less bathroom I had to worry about. That made things better for me, but he really didn't like it at all.

The first time he tried to get into the bedroom and it was locked, he was really surprised. After that, he'd go to the door and try to get in. When he couldn't open it, he'd knock, and then he'd start to pound on it. After a while, he'd come back down the hall and look at me and say, "Damn it, she's got the damned door locked again." It was as if he were talking to someone else, like we had a third person in the house. I'd ask him why he needed to go in there, but he didn't know.

Right in the middle of all the bizarre behaviors, Howdy had six good days in a row with hardly any incidents at all. So, when he started to act up again, I really let it get to me. Why did I let it bother me at all? When we had so many peaceful days, I guess I didn't expect them to end - I allowed myself to believe he might become normal again.

One particular Tuesday started out really well. However, before lunch, Howdy managed to urinate in the wastebasket, and then dump coffee grounds all over the living room rug. I no sooner got that mess cleaned up when he turned the hose on in the driveway. By the time I got the hose turned off, Howdy had let all of the bleach water out of the sink in the shed I had our white clothes soaking in. Later on, Howdy kept taking his slippers on and off, and complaining about his feet hurting. I finally decided to check, and sure enough, he had a bunch of toilet tissue stuffed in the toes of his slippers.

All in all, I thought it took an awfully long time to get the Cogentin out of his system. Howdy continued to have bad days long after the "week from hell." One of the more amusing incidents during that period involved Howdy misplacing his teeth. He'd always blame me when he couldn't find them. One day, after I gave him some peanuts and they got stuck under his upper plate, he took his teeth out of his mouth and threw them into the bathroom rubbish can – once again, it was my fault. When he became angry with me, he wouldn't do anything I asked him to do. Whenever that happened, I knew there wouldn't be any sleep that night, and I was right. Even if I gave him a sleeping pill, he wouldn't go to sleep. The only good thing about having a week of bad days was the hope that more good days were ahead.

CHAPTER 9 – FOOT PROBLEMS

Howdy had a history of problems with his feet. He'd been going to a podiatrist on a regular basis most of his life. He had a hammertoe, and severely ingrown toenails, which were very painful. He also had very bad calluses and trouble with his arches. At one time, he even had a spur on his heel, which was also very painful. Howdy was a baker his entire adult life, so he stood on his feet for long, hard hours, and the concrete floors were very hard on his feet.

Howdy visited a podiatrist about every three to five months. Those trips were always prompted by his inability to endure the pain any longer. He never seemed to mind going to the podiatrist, and I always figured that was because the podiatrist gave him relief from the pain. When Howdy's ingrown nails started curling in more and more, I knew he was in a lot of pain just by the way he walked.

I never had problems with my feet, but my mother did. I vividly remembered how much she suffered, and how she'd break into tears after a day of standing on her feet with the pain being almost unbearable. Because of my having gone through all that with my mother, I had a great deal of sympathy for what Howdy was going through. On one visit in 1985, the podiatrist explained to me that he could relieve Howdy of a great deal of his pain by performing a minor surgical procedure on his feet. I told him to go ahead and set it up.

I had no idea the operation would further complicate our lives by creating other problems. After I spoke with the podiatrist, I tried to explain things to Howdy, but he just couldn't understand. I talked to him, and tried to tell him what was wrong with his feet, and what had to be done about it. But he just grinned that childlike grin I loved so much and I knew he had no idea what I was trying to tell him.

On a Friday, I took Howdy to an ambulatory care center in Tampa for pre-operation tests. The ordeal began with a major struggle to get Howdy out of bed early on the morning we were to go to the clinic. As luck would have it, Howdy was in a deep slumber when it came time to wake up, and I had a terrible time getting him awake and ready to go. Finally, I managed to get him dressed and into the car, and off we went.

The drive to Tampa was uneventful and I was grateful for that. When we arrived at the clinic, a nurse gave Howdy a small bottle for a urine sample. She escorted him to a restroom and explained what he needed to do. When he came out, he'd filled the bottle up with water. So, I had to go into the restroom with him and we did it the right way. That gave everyone a big laugh – at least some things could still be funny.

Thereafter, things went smoothly until it was time for X-rays. We were able to get Howdy into the X-ray room, and on the table okay, but he made it quite clear he wasn't going to stay there without me. After considering the alternatives, the nurse decided I could be in the room with him. They put me behind a screen, but Howdy had to see me, or he wouldn't stay on the table. So I went back and forth from the table to behind the curtain. It took a while, but we finally made it through the X-rays. They showed them to me, and explained what needed to be done. They were planning to cut off all of his ingrown nails, except the one on his hammertoe. To fix the hammertoe, the doctor would be cutting away part of the bone, and to minimize the risk of infection, the nail would have to stay. The doctor and I were both worried about infection. We decided to proceed, so the doctor sent us home until the operation could be scheduled. Other than the problem with taking the X-rays, everything went pretty well, and the trip home was uneventful.

We scheduled the operation for October. Again, we had to go back to Tampa for the surgery, which I was prepared for, but I was not prepared for what was to follow. Even the doctor didn't realize the problems that would ensue.

The operation went smoothly, but the aftermath turned into a real mess. Howdy was bandaged heavily as we headed for home with a fistful of prescriptions I had to get filled. We stopped at Herbert and Sylvia's house, and I asked them if they could stay with him at our place while I went for the prescriptions. They agreed to help me out, but they'd never been alone with Howdy since he'd become so belligerent. Unfortunately, it never occurred to me with Howdy just having gone through such a traumatic experience, plus me not being there, he'd be even more agitated than normal.

While I was waiting for the prescriptions to be filled at the pharmacy, the phone rang. It was for me. Herbert called to say they were having a hard time with Howdy, and could I get home as soon as possible. Fortunately, the prescriptions were ready, so I rushed home.

First of all, Howdy didn't like having bandages on. Then, on top of that, seeing all that blood must have upset him a great deal. Also, the medicine was wearing off, and I'm sure he was in a lot of pain. Later, Herbert and Sylvia told me Howdy went to the bathroom, and ripped off half of the bandages shortly after I left for the drugstore. Then he came into the living room, and started taking the rest of the bandages off, and they were afraid to try to stop him because he was in such an enraged state.

What a mess! By the time I got home, Howdy had pulled off all the bandages, and there was blood everywhere. My first concern was the potential for infection because he was walking on the dirty carpet.

Prior to that moment, I'd been doing a pretty good job of keeping my emotions in check, but I just lost it and got hysterical again. I called the podiatrist, and he calmed me down by telling me what to do to make everything all right again. He'd been through Alzheimer's with his father, so he knew what I was going through more than any other doctor I'd encountered up to that time. He told me there were more good days than bad, and sometimes just by putting it out of my mind overnight, it'd all seem trivial in the morning. His willingness to take the time to reassure me worked wonders for my outlook.

The healing process continued for over a month. Fortunately, Howdy didn't develop an infection in his foot. But it was very hard keeping bandages on him, so we went through a lot of bandages and tape.

After that incident with Herbert and Sylvia, it became apparent not everyone could handle someone with Alzheimer's. You just can't bring someone in to take care of an Alzheimer's patient if they don't understand all the complexities of the disease. From that point on, I decided I couldn't leave him with anyone until much later when he was unable to get around.

In December of 1985, I noticed Howdy was getting very shaky - even more than usual. When he tried to lift his cup of coffee to take a drink, he couldn't tilt it far enough to get it to his lips. That represented another big change in him. I could only wonder, "What would be next?"

Right after that, Howdy reverted to his constant restlessness once again. Along with the restlessness, he was also busy getting into mischief again. But this time, he began to nap a lot more than usual. I guessed all that activity wore him out. No wonder he was so tired - he moved almost constantly.

One day Howdy asked me, "Where's the wood?"

"We don't have any," I replied. "What do you want wood for anyway?"

"I want to build a fire in the living room because it's getting cold," he said.

"It's 90 degrees!" I explained. "Where are you planning on building this fire?"

He pointed to the middle of the living room.

"How are you going to build a fire, we don't have a fireplace," I told him.

He thought about it for a minute, and then he decided it was pretty funny, and we both had a big laugh.

Another day, he suddenly had an inordinate interest in the stereo. It seemed as if he wanted to play with it by turning the dials over and over. After I finally convinced him to leave it alone, he went into the bedroom and came out about ten minutes later with one of my blouses on and two of his belts. He also had his watch on his ankle. I told him he looked funny, and asked him where he was going. He answered, "Why, outside, of course!" After I told him he looked silly, we both giggled about his foolishness.

After our shower one morning, I decided to sit in the dressing room and watch how Howdy did things. First he put shaving cream on his face, and then he washed it off. Then he started to shave. After I convinced him to reapply the shave cream, he finished shaving. He followed the shave by putting his deodorant on his face instead of his after-shave lotion. Then I handed him his underwear and shirt and left him for a few minutes. When I returned, his shorts were on backward and his legs were in his shirtsleeves. He also had his glasses on upside down. We spent a lot of time rearranging things he disarranged. It kept us both quite busy.

About that time, Howdy began not letting me put his pills in his mouth. So I tried getting around that by putting them in his hand, and when I wasn't looking he put them in lots of different places. I found them in the toilet, in the plants, in the sink, even in his pockets.

Howdy reached the point where he knew the eating utensils were used for something, "But what?" He'd pick up his straw, and after looking at it for a long time, he'd try to use it as a fork. When he couldn't manage the food, his anger would boil over. Either he'd bang on the counter, or he'd throw his food across the room. Those were extremely trying times for both of us. It always bothered me when I'd see how hurt he became when he realized what he'd done. I just couldn't imagine the feeling of frustration he must have been going through.

I decided it was time to schedule another visit with Dr. Hughes, as much for me to have a talk with the doctor about my mental health, as for him to examine Howdy.

December 20, 1985:

History and physical: he is stable on Haldol i mg b.i.d., he is terribly confused. He's had one incidence of fecal incontinence, but it's not a problem. The disease traumatizes his wife. We had a long talk with her today.

Physical exam: He has a wet cough, his lungs sound ok, but he obviously has bronchitis. Afebrils, heart sounds normal, he is totally disoriented.

Assessment: Bronchitis. OBS.

Plan: I put him on Amoxil 250 t.i.d. x 10 days, I'll see him reg.

In the beginning, the incontinence would come and go, and since Howdy was unhappy with Pampers, we took a lot of chances going without them. But I had to learn to put pads everywhere. That seemed to work out pretty well. Through the years, I improved at finding good solutions for various situations that cropped up.

During our visit to Dr. Hughes, he asked us to follow him into the examining room. When the doctor turned around and asked me, "How's the dummy?" I was so astounded I couldn't respond. To this day, I can't figure out why I let him get away with saying that. Even though he was kidding, I'll never forget it.

Whenever Howdy slept for longer periods, I had to be busy. It never mattered what I did, just as long as I was busy. I loved painting, so I painted furniture, porch floors, and anything else that needed painting, to occupy my mind and my hands. Most of it was spray painting, but even using a brush was something I loved to do. I actually got quite good with a can of spray paint. Also, while we were in Florida, I'd mow our yard and both of our neighbors' yards. They were still up north during the summer months. That was in the early years before we started going up north for longer periods ourselves.

We made it to the year 1986, but not without our share of trials and tribulations. Each year things seemed to get a little worse. Since I was still having trouble handling my own feelings, how did I expect others to react to Howdy?

Sometime later, Sylvia told me she didn't think she could care for someone the way I cared for Howdy. But until you're faced with a loved one in a circumstance like that, you never know what you're capable of doing. One of our neighbors told me God doesn't give you anything you can't handle. Thereafter, I tried to let that be my motto.

As Howdy lost more and more of his abilities, people told me I needed to get "Power of Attorney" as I'd eventually have to sign for everything. That was a big decision for me because it meant Howdy was never going to get well again. For some reason, I didn't want to admit that. Finally, we went to an attorney, and it turned out Howdy was barely able to sign the papers. I'm sure if we had waited another month or two, it would've been too late.

CHAPTER 10 – A HOME IN OHIO AND FLORIDA

The worse Howdy got, the more I thought about moving back to Ohio. We were just too far away from our family. I reasoned that as future emergencies came up, the distance factor was going to play a large part in how we'd be able to deal with those emergencies. I knew my sister, Mary Jane, and her husband, Jess, would never be able to make the trip to Florida from Pennsylvania as often as they could come to Ohio if I needed their help. And little did I imagine then how desperately I'd need their assistance in the years ahead.

Also, the trip from Florida to Ohio, and back, was becoming very hard on Howdy and me. We were beginning to make that 20-hour trip back and forth without stopping overnight at a motel. If we ran into bad weather, how long would it take me to get Howdy out of the car and into a motel? Was it better to get him soaked and take the chance of him getting pneumonia, or drive straight through? So I decided to keep on driving, stopping only for hot coffee, food, and restroom breaks. As tortuous as it might sound, it really wasn't too bad, and the coffee seemed to perk me up.

I knew Howdy would only worsen as each year went by, and that helped me make the decision to consider buying a place in Ohio where we could live for half the year. At the time, the help we received in Florida was very limited. Since I didn't know what was in store for us, I really didn't know how much help we'd need. Moving to Ohio turned out to be the best decision I ever made. But, leaving our friends in Florida, even for part of the year, was quite difficult.

So, when we drove back to Ohio in the spring of 1986, I was pretty sure I'd end up looking for a place to live up there. Once we "moved in" with John and his family, and I saw how crowded we all were in that little house, I made up my mind that looking for a place of our own in Delaware was essential. Since we couldn't afford to spend too much money, imagine my surprise, while shopping one day, to see six or eight mobile homes sitting on a vacant lot. In front of the homes was a big sign stating that the owners were opening a new mobile home park in Delaware.

I decided to stop and look, and after we talked for a while, the salesman took us for a ride to where they'd started the park. There were only about five or six homes already sitting on lots, so as an added incentive, we had our pick of the best lots.

After much deliberation and soul searching, I settled on the lot nearest to the mailboxes. There was a deep ravine behind several of the other lots, and knowing how much Howdy liked to roam, I felt safer with a flat lot. Another consideration was with us being in Florida at least half of the year, and the mobile home park not being in the best part of town, our trailer would be more secure in a highly visible location.

The next challenge was to find just the right mobile home. I settled on a single-wide, with two bedrooms and two baths - one bedroom and a bath at each end of the mobile home. The kitchen, laundry area, and living room were in the center of the house. It came furnished, so we didn't need any of our Florida furniture. I figured we could always leave our furniture in Florida, if and when we decided to go north permanently, and that would be a good selling point. All we needed to do in order to move into the new house, and begin living there, was buy dishes, pots and pans, towels, and kitchenware. I loved the home and the location, so it didn't take much talking for me to decide to buy (even though I was the one who had to make all the decisions, I liked to think I had Howdy's unspoken approval for all the decisions I made). Once we signed the papers, we just had to wait for the home to be moved onto the lot, and we were able to take possession.

Within a few days, the home was ready and we moved in. From that time forward, we had much more time for our family, and when Mary Jane and Jess wanted to visit us, we had enough room to put them up. John, Betsy, John Howard, and Janean also had their house to themselves again, and we were just a few minutes away whenever we wanted to visit – it was truly the best of all worlds!

The home itself was 14 feet wide by 70 feet long, so with the way it was situated on the lot, the side, or length of the trailer, faced the street. I really liked that because it gave the trailer a distinctive look since almost all the other homes in the park were perpendicular to the street. We had a nice long, wide roof put over the patio, which was located on the front and ran about half the length of the house. The patio was about 30 feet long and in the spring and summer it became our lookout to the world. It was especially nice for Howdy because he could sit out there and enjoy the view as the people passed by.

Almost immediately, I fell in love with the mobile home and the park. After we got settled in, I had quite a job of landscaping to do, and I relished the challenge of making our home the loveliest in the park. Soon, we had to put up a shed to hold all of our tools, the lawn mower, etc. We even had enough of a yard to put in a few trees for shade. Since Delaware has many flowering crabapple trees, I decided to put two on our lot as well. Digging in the dirt was one of my favorite jobs. I went hog wild with the planting. That first summer, I put in several double clematis vines, lots of flowers, and I even put in a small bush and carved a topiary in the shape of six balls. I'm proud to say I was able to keep it in good shape all the years we lived there.

Even with the distraction of settling into a new home, Howdy's behavior patterns were just as unpredictable in Ohio as they'd been in Florida. One day, shortly after we moved in, he called to me from outside. He was having trouble trying to figure out how to come into the house. I had to go out and show him how to come up the stairs and turn the knob to open the door. He was so tired after that ordeal I put him to bed for a nap at 2:45. It turned out to be a short nap, as he was awake by 2:55. I put him back down again at 3:00. This time, he slept until 4:00. There were many days when I was thankful he even took a nap. No matter what else was going on, there were bound to be new experiences almost every day.

For example, Howdy suddenly started having trouble when he got up at night to go to the bathroom. He seemed to have difficulty walking straight ahead, so he'd stagger to his right and almost fall down. One night he started to fall, and knowing I couldn't carry him, I caught him and gently leaned him toward the bed and he landed on the bed instead of the floor. Many times, however, when he fell, I couldn't get to him in time, and he did fall on the floor. Once he was down there, I had an awful time trying to lift him up off the floor. I now believe all that strenuous activity triggered my asthma, which became more and more of a problem for me as the years of caring for Howdy wore on. Even that summer of 1986, while the asthma wasn't too bad, there were times when it'd be impossible for me to hoist him up from the floor because of my difficulty breathing. Sometimes my lungs felt as if they were going to burst. Then I'd begin coughing, and I couldn't do anything. When it became impossible for me to get Howdy back on his feet, I had to get help. If someone from the family wasn't available, I'd dial 911 and the rescuers were always there in a few minutes. I can't imagine what we'd have done without them.

Another example of an inexplicable change in Howdy's behavior concerned his sleeping habits. For a long time, Howdy slept on his back. There were a couple of years when he never turned on his side at all while he was sleeping. So, when he half turned on his side one night, I was surprised. I always wondered what caused those types of changes. Why did he suddenly turn over on his side? Had he slept that way several times per week, I don't think I'd have given it another thought.

As we progressed through the summer of 1986, I began to adjust to living in Delaware once again, and I gradually felt less stress. My whole outlook changed in a positive way. The things that happened were just as odd, but I found myself better able to cope with the increasingly difficult circumstances. I found myself reacting in a much calmer way. Maybe I was becoming accustomed to the changes.

One day, out of the blue, Howdy wanted to touch me again, not with passion, but with a tenderness I remembered so well. For years, he didn't seem to care. Those were the times when I fantasized he might get well again.

One night, while we were in bed, Howdy got cold. He reached over and pulled a blanket over me. I guess he figured I must be have been cold, too.

On some nights, Howdy went to bed all by himself. Evidently, he just got tired, so he toddled off the way he used to. There were also times when I saw him watching TV, and laughing the way he had in the past. So many times, little encouraging signs like those raised my hopes he was going to recover - especially when those "normal" episodes lasted longer than usual. But, subconsciously, despite what I felt in my heart, I knew it just couldn't be.

I didn't give Howdy sleeping pills every day, only when he became too aggressive. I didn't want to make a zombie out of him. When I told him I loved him and hugged him, I wanted him to know I still truly cared for him. I can't say how many times I did that each day. And even though he didn't always react in an obvious way, I knew he understood. Just to see that smile on his face was reward enough.

I always loved it when we'd have company, because with Howdy's deteriorating condition, I was less and less able to leave the house. Unfortunately, having company also had its negative side. Whenever our friends stayed for a few days, Howdy went through some bad times after they left. I never knew if that was his way of showing disappointment because they were gone, or if he simply needed to hear the sound of other people's voices, and have the companionship of other people. The change in Howdy was always temporary, thank goodness, and after a while, he'd always be himself again.

On one such occasion, Howdy got out of bed in the morning and proceeded to make the bed. He then ate a good breakfast, and I didn't have to help him with it at all. He seemed so alert. He even sat in front of the TV, and actually started laughing at the humorous situations on the show we had on. Then he went to the bathroom all by himself. What a pleasant surprise! Later, he wanted to change his shirt in the living room. Unfortunately, he wanted to pull the shirt over his head as he stood under the fan, which was on at the time. I was afraid he'd get his hands caught in the fan, so I helped him at that point. But, for a few glorious hours, it was as if I had my Howdy back, and everything was right with the world once again.

When we went through good times like that, life was so effortless. I'd almost forget all of the bad times. I could never understand the ups and downs of Alzheimer's. There were other days, for example, when Howdy could read as well as he ever did. When that happened, it seemed as if he had to read everything he got his hands on. Not only did he feel compelled to read everything, but also for some reason, he had to read it to me out loud.

I also couldn't get over the change in Howdy whenever our son, John, came over for a visit. I could never figure out if John just always said and did things that made Howdy laugh, or whether there was something about his voice. Howdy always perked up the minute John walked through the door. I guess there's really something to that old adage, "we all need laughter in our lives." Howdy was certainly proof of that, because he always seemed much calmer and brighter when he was laughing. And John certainly knew how to make him laugh.

I noticed, too, Howdy seemed to be in a much better mood when he was around other people. I figured he got tired of me telling him what to do and what not to do all the time. I also assumed there were times when he thought I was a bit bossy, but I was the one who had to tell him what he could and couldn't do. That's not to say we didn't find lots of things to share a laugh about. We had a lot of fun times, and I was always grateful Howdy and I got along so well together and, all considered, we had many more good times than bad. I tried my best, most of the time, to make everything seem funny, hoping that would make him feel better. And it worked more often than not.

After spending more time in Ohio than we'd originally planned that summer, it was time to begin packing for the long trip back to Florida. It was late in September, and the cold weather would soon be upon us. When it came time to go, we were always torn between thoughts of leaving our family, and getting to be with our good friends in Florida again. Of course, I already knew, sooner or later, we'd be spending all of our time in Ohio.

CHAPTER 11 – UPS AND DOWNS

It seemed as if the trip back and forth became more difficult with each passing year – on both of us. I was becoming weary of all the housecleaning involved at each location when we closed one home to go to the other one. There were walls to be washed and curtains to be cleaned and re-hung. The venetian blinds were a big pain in the neck. It got to the point that I really hated venetian blinds. No matter how hard I worked to get things ready, I never got everything done before it was time for us to leave.

Once again, we made that long, exhausting trip back to Dade City. And once again, I was very grateful that we made it without too much trouble along the way. When we arrived back home in Florida, or Ohio, there were always lots of things that needed to be done at that end, too. First, I had to unpack the car. Even though we only had travel necessities and clothing to cart back and forth, it got to be quite a chore. Next, I'd go to the store with a long list of food we'd need right away. When that was done, and I had time to look around, everything looked as if it had an inch thick covering of dust. So, I spent a couple days just dusting. Then all of the dishes, and pots and pans had to be washed after they sat unused for so long. Every once in a while, I felt like the ceilings, walls, or something else needed painting, too. So, I'd go out and buy the paint and get to work on that project. It got to the point, where I felt like all I did was clean house at both locations.

We had to leave chemicals in the Florida house when we went away because of the bugs. So, I had to give the house a good airing out after we returned. It's no wonder I ended up with asthma and related breathing problems. Even the cleaning products started to bother me about that time.

Once we settled back into our normal routine in Florida in the fall of 1986, it seemed as if keeping an eye on Howdy was even more of a job than it'd been before. Even though I had to work harder to watch Howdy's every move, he became more lovable as his condition continued to deteriorate. As Howdy became more dependent on me, I loved him all the more.

A few nights after our arrival back in Florida, I thought Howdy was ready to go to sleep, so I put him to bed. Imagine my surprise when a half-hour later he came into the living room and said, "She was here."

I asked him, "Who was here?"

"Your mother and she told me what I could do." Then he said in a loud voice, **"The hell with that business!"**

After calming him down, I put him back in bed. About 11:00 P.M., he woke up again, came into the living room, and asked me where **his** mother was. I knew right away we were in for another bad night. He came out of the bedroom almost every hour that evening, and each time, he asked me a question, or made a statement, as he did earlier. Before I answered him, I made sure I gave his question considerable thought, so I didn't make him angry again.

Normally, when he had trouble sleeping, he wouldn't stay in bed. I think he needed to be near someone. I always asked him what was wrong, or did he need anything? Sometimes he'd say he wanted to hug me. He'd just stand in one place until I gave him a few hugs and kisses. When I told him I loved him, it seemed to relax and comfort him. Sometimes, I'd get into bed beside him and hug him and that calmed him enough to fall asleep. But, that didn't mean he'd stay sleeping.

Sleep for Howdy was virtually impossible when I couldn't figure out a way to get him to relax. It got to the point where Howdy was constantly restless, not only during the daytime, but all night, too. He seemed to be in constant motion. Not gentle movements, but terrible thrashing during which the whole bed shook. Then he'd moan and groan like he was in terrible pain. It was nothing for him to fall out of bed several times each night. On one of those nights, I just couldn't get him back in bed. So, I propped him up with several pillows surrounding him on the floor. Even then, he kept rolling around with his knees going up and down repeatedly. By morning, he had some of the worst rug burns I ever saw, and I felt awful I hadn't been able to get him back in bed.

That's when I decided I had to come up with a plan to keep him from hurting himself when he fell out of bed. So, the next morning, I took a mattress off a trundle bed we had, and put it on his side of the bed on the floor. That seemed to work out pretty well. At least he didn't have so far to fall, and from that point on, when he did fall out of bed, he landed on the mattress and no damage was done.

On another night, when I thought I had everything secured, I put him to bed and decided to play backgammon. I settled into a good game, when all of a sudden, I heard Howdy grunting and groaning. I raced to the bedroom to investigate. Howdy had fallen out of bed and had somehow managed to wedge his leg and his arm between the bed rail and the mattress. It was like trying to put together a huge jigsaw puzzle as I struggled to get him untangled. I don't know which one of us laughed the most. Finally, I got him back into bed, and returned to my game.

I hardly had time to sit down before he was moaning again. I ran into the bedroom only to find Howdy back on the floor. In that short space of time, he'd somehow wiggled to the door. There he was - half in, and half out, of the doorway. Try as I might, I couldn't budge him. So, I put a pillow under his head and a blanket over him. Then I placed my chair so I could watch him for the rest of the night. When I decided to go to bed that evening, I curled up on the floor beside him, and that's the way we spent the remainder of the night.

Many of our challenges involved ordinary, everyday activities that suddenly became a mystery to Howdy. Just a simple thing like being able to put his coffee cup to his mouth, or being able to drink from a glass with a straw became a challenge. Those simple tasks became major projects as time went on. But whenever he did an activity correctly, he always knew he'd done something great. Afterwards, he'd sit there with a big grin on his face and wait for me to praise him.

Then there were the times when Howdy did a task correctly, but maybe not at the correct time. For example, every so often, Howdy would insist on putting his hat on his head before he went to bed. He had no problem putting the hat on the right way. When I looked in on him later, sure enough, he was still wearing his hat. He really liked wearing a hat.

An old friend of ours came for a visit one day, and Howdy remembered her. For some unexplainable reason, his mental abilities and his behaviors were always better when there were other people around. That day, he was able to pull his chair closer to the table without any help from me. He even asked for more food, which was unusual. From time to time, he looked at his watch, and then told her what time it was - and it was the correct time. When he perked up like that, I never knew if he was just showing off, or if he needed someone's approval. Our friend decided to test Howdy, so she held up two magazines. He read the names on both of them correctly.

After our friend left, Howdy was depressed for several hours. Then all of a sudden, he snapped out of it and was smiling again. The more I write these remembrances, the more I realize the patterns Howdy fell into repeated themselves over and over.

While we were in Ohio the previous summer, Howdy's doctor had put him on a different sleeping pill. Those pills must have been quite powerful, because he'd sleep anywhere from 12 to 15 hours after taking one of the pills. I began to wonder if the pharmacy in Dade City was giving him generic pills that weren't as strong as the ones he'd been taking up north. Again, I was clutching at straws looking for explanations to quell my doubts and fears. Ten minutes after taking one of the pills we brought with us from Ohio, Howdy was out like a light. But I could never be sure Howdy would react to the pills the same way every time. Howdy either didn't sleep very much at all, or he slept much longer than he should have. When he did sleep, it was a very, deep sleep. He usually didn't move around much while he was in one of those pill-induced deep slumbers, either. I'd go into the bedroom to check up on him frequently. I'd listen to make sure he was still breathing normally, and sometimes I'd just watch him sleep. He looked so peaceful you'd never know there was anything wrong with him. Occasionally, however, he'd sleep for up to 20 hours, and that's when I'd start to worry about him. I'd check on him even more often than I usually did, but he always seemed to be breathing normally. So, I'd find myself sitting in my chair watching the clock to see how long it'd been since the last time I checked on him.

On another day, Howdy strolled around the room several times while I was sitting in my chair. All of a sudden, he stopped in front of me and gestured for me to get up. When I did, he sat down in my chair and giggled as if he'd just performed a great feat of trickery. Quite often, I reflected on how Howdy's behaviors were increasingly childlike as his condition worsened.

At one point, Howdy went 41 straight days without a sleeping pill, and he was on his best behavior the whole time. It was great for me. That represented another happy time in our lives, when I thought he was going to get better. It was truly fun while it lasted.

Another time, after Howdy had gone through two great days, he was confused and disoriented and generally out of it, when he got up the next morning. He started the day off by putting his under shorts in the toilet. I asked him why he did that, and he said, "What was I supposed to do with them? They were dirty."

So, I asked him if he wanted me to help him finish dressing. He said, "No, I can do it!" When he got obstinate like that, I'd wait until he decided he couldn't do it by himself, and then I'd give him a hand. I was actually pleased he always wanted to be fully clothed, at least until he became bedridden. Howdy always checked himself out in a mirror after he got dressed, and he usually seemed happy with what he saw.

Sometimes, when I'd leave him by himself to get dressed, he'd come out of the bedroom with one sock on and no shoes. If he came out with everything on the right way, it was a big plus for the day.

One morning, after we had a hassle getting him ready for the day, I expected him to be really hungry. I told him to come eat breakfast. He said he didn't feel hungry. So I thought we'd dispense with breakfast that day. But less than two minutes later, he spied a pom-pom with a bright ribbon wrapped around it. He began to eat the ribbon. In order to get the ribbon away from him, I told him I'd replace it with a waffle. He thought about it for a minute, and decided it sounded like a good idea and ate the waffle instead.

That same night, he fell out of bed again. I was at wits end because I didn't want him sleeping on the floor all the time, but I also didn't want him to hurt himself. I even thought about putting sides on the bed. But I was afraid he'd somehow get tangled in whatever we'd use for sides. So, I went back to putting a mattress on the floor, or sometimes I'd just use a lot of pillows. Once again, we were in a mode that if he fell out of bed again, there'd be less chance of him getting hurt.

A few days later, Howdy went through another period of nonstop activity whenever he was awake. Day after day he just couldn't sit down. He was constantly moving the furniture from one place to another, and rolling the kitchen rugs all up and putting them in the living room.

When the furniture moving got boring, he decided he needed someone to talk to. I watched him as he went to the wall where I had a number of family pictures hanging. He took down one of the pictures of me and began talking to it. Tiring of that, he started whistling, and then he told some invisible someone to, "Get over here!" Suddenly, he looked up and spotted himself in the mirror, so he started talking to his image. It was definitely a one-sided conversation.

On another day, I found Howdy rubbing his eyebrows over and over, and then he started rubbing his eyes. I asked him if they were sore and he said, "Yes." I asked him if he wanted me to put a warm towel on his eyes and he said, "Yes, that would be very nice." After changing the towel several times he seemed to be better, so we took it off. Never again did he have that same problem.

CHAPTER 12 – FRIENDS IN NEED, FRIENDS INDEED

Howdy's struggles with incontinence continued into 1986, and as the year went on, it became more and more of a problem for us to deal with. It happened so seldom in the beginning I wasn't prepared for it. Howdy still objected to wearing pads of any kind, so when he had a BM it bothered him a great deal. I'm sure he didn't know what was happening. But when it did happen, everything got soiled - floor, bed sheets, long pants, underwear, carpets, furniture – everything. The fact that I took it so calmly was a miracle in itself. In the final analysis, it simply came down to me feeling sorrier for Howdy than I did for myself. The terribly devastated look on his face was enough to tear my heart out. The worse Howdy became, the more I loved him. I don't know why, but that's the way it was.

The incontinence actually began in Florida before we went north for the summer. Even though it could be quite a problem for me to deal with, I never seemed to be prepared for it, because Howdy would sometimes go weeks without an incident. It didn't seem to matter where he was at, when the urge struck him, we had a mess. Then I'd clean it up again until the next episode.

After our long stay in Ohio, and all the time it took us to get settled back into our Florida home, I realized it had been quite a while since Howdy visited Dr. Hughes. So, I called the doctor's office and made an appointment. I felt Howdy needed to be seen by his doctors on a regular basis, because we never knew what would come up next. I always made a point of telling Howdy it was time to visit the doctor again, so it didn't come as a surprise.

October 8, 1986:

History and physical: his OBS is deteriorated somewhat, they're controlling him with small doses of Haldol, which is making some slight difference in his condition. Otherwise, no medical problems, he was not hospitalized this past summer while he was in Ohio.

Exam: he looks pretty good, totally disoriented. His BP is 122/80, lungs clear, heart sounds normal.

Assessment OBS.

Plan: His wife has him pretty stable, we'll leave him as is.

Howdy had a strong heart, liver, bladder and most of his organs were good, but his lungs would eventually give him trouble.

Even as his condition worsened, Howdy loved going shopping. Consequently, we went on shopping excursions as often as I felt up to it. Many times, we went to a large shopping mall in Lakeland with our friends, Ethel and Jim Smith. Ethel and I always left the men on a bench when we went into one of the stores. Then we'd move on to another store and the men moved to another bench, and then another, and another. We'd keep shopping until one, or all of us, began to tire. After we wore ourselves out, we liked to pick out a nice restaurant and have a pleasant lunch. Then we'd get into the car and head for home, usually very satisfied with how the day had gone, and how well Howdy had done.

As the months passed, and Howdy's condition continued to deteriorate, it was so gratifying our friends stuck with us. I came to enjoy the company of other people even more than I had before, and I truly cherished the conversations we had – all of that was essential to my well being. I think we all looked forward to those times together.

Before Howdy became too ill, sometimes we'd get together with two other couples –six being the number we could cram into one of our cars - and take short sightseeing trips together. Other times, we'd just go out to eat together at a restaurant somewhere. On those occasions when we were all together, it was like one, big, happy family. It was as if Howdy belonged to all of them. No matter who was sitting next to Howdy, they'd take care of him, like putting his napkin on, or cutting up his meat. The men never hesitated to offer to take him to the restroom, either. Howdy was our top priority.

When it became too difficult for me to handle Howdy in someone else's home, we decided it'd be easier to have everyone come to our house. By doing it that way, we found we could get together more often. And that was just fine with me.

Everyone met at our house and each couple brought part of the meal. After dinner, the women always gathered in the kitchen, and amid much laughter, cleaned up. The men gathered in the living room with Howdy and watched TV. First they watched the news, then Jeopardy, and, of course, Wheel Of Fortune. Usually, by the time Jeopardy was on, the women had completed washing and drying the dishes, so we joined the men. It was always amazing to me what women can find to talk and laugh about while doing dishes. My, how the time flew by.

Most of those evenings, usually during Jeopardy, I'd put Howdy to bed with the fervent hope he'd be in for the night. There were times when he did stay in bed for the whole night, but other nights, I'd be kept busy going back and forth to take care of him.

At eight o'clock, we always made a mad dash for the dining room table and out came the cards, or dice, or dominoes for a fun-filled evening of games. If we were playing cards and Howdy woke up, someone always played my hand for me while I was gone. About 10:30, we usually put on the coffeepot, and started cutting the cake, or pie, to top off the evening. We usually broke up about 11:00 or 12:00, and oh, how I hated to see the evening end. With hugs and kisses we all said goodnight.

The days when everyone came over to play shuffleboard on the courts at the end of our street were much longer, and I have fond memories of those days. Howdy and I played as long as we could, but eventually, we had to quit because Howdy didn't understand what to do.

Thereafter, our friends stopped at our house on the way to the courts to drop off whatever they'd brought for the evening meal and snacking. After they finished playing, they all came to our house for the rest of the day. Then we started playing cards, board games, dice, or whatever diversion everyone agreed upon.

We always seemed to be having so much fun we hated to stop to eat, but retired people do like to eat. Those days were much too short, even though they lasted till eleven or so.

My biggest regret, when we were forced to move from Florida to Ohio permanently, was leaving all those wonderful people behind. For years we went to each other's houses, for a good meal, pleasant conversation, TV watching, playing cards, playing games, or for a good game of Dominos. I wish I had it all to do over again, because I'd love to do it all again. Friendship is certainly one of the greatest gifts you can possibly have.

Of course, we weren't always with our friends, and when Howdy and I were alone, we still had our little challenges to face. Part of our normal routine was for us to do our grocery shopping at our local Wynn-Dixie store. We'd always enter the store and go to a bench located at the front, near the cash registers. After getting Howdy comfortably seated, I'd get a cart and tell him to stay put while I shopped. That worked out quite well until one day, when I got back to the checkout counter and Howdy was nowhere in sight. Talk about panic. Even though Howdy had two I.D. bracelets (one for Ohio and one for Florida) on his wrist, I still worried about what would happen to him if he got lost. As soon as someone you know becomes forgetful and starts to wander off, get an ID bracelet and somehow convince them they have to wear it - even if you have to put it on their ankle, or even on a chain around their neck. At least, if they wander off, they can be identified and you'll be notified where they're at.

When I realized Howdy had wondered off that day, I went to the office. The people in that store knew us because we shopped there all the time, so they knew Howdy had Alzheimer's, and they were very helpful and concerned. The manager immediately sent one of the boys to the men's restroom, but Howdy wasn't in there. Then he sent a couple of boys out to the parking lot, but they couldn't find him out there, either.

Once we had exhausted all of those possibilities, I **really** panicked. Frantically, I set off to each of the stores in the shopping center to see if I could find him. After searching several stores near the super market, I decided to go to the other end of the shopping center to the hardware store. I remembered something had caught his eye the last time we were in there, so I figured it was worth a try. Sure enough, there he was, and was he ever glad to see me. I was so relieved, but I also remembered the concern of everyone in Wynn-Dixie. I made a point of taking him back there so they'd know he was safe. Everyone was genuinely pleased to know he was okay, and several of them shook his hand and told him to be careful. I think each time we visited that store thereafter everyone kept one eye on Howdy till we left.

On another shopping trip, we'd just entered a store when one of the cashiers came over to me, and asked if I minded if she gave me a kiss and a hug. Naturally, I was a little taken aback, but I said, "Okay." While she was hugging me, she said she'd been watching us for a long time and just felt she had to tell me how great she thought I was for the good care I gave Howdy.

Wow! I just can't tell you what a tremendous boost that was for my morale. I think all of us need a little praise every once in a while. I received a good lesson about the compassion of others. It sure helped to restore my faith in humanity - people really do care.

At that time, I'd have appreciated it if Howdy's neurologist had been as observant as that cashier, and had given me some credit for the care I was giving Howdy instead of telling me to, "Calm down, and take care of your husband!" I must say Doctor Hughes was always good about telling me how nice Howdy looked, and what a good job I was doing taking care of him.

Christmas seemed to come around quickly that year and we all appreciated being together during the Holidays. Harry was with us again. A few months earlier his son and his family moved to Tennessee, so Harry sold his house in Michigan in September. Then he moved to Aliquippa, Pennsylvania to be near Mary Jane and her family. Thereafter, he lived in Pennsylvania during the summer and with us in Florida in the winter. Since we all were away from our families, we did our best to make the holidays a happy occasion. One way we could do that was to buy each other some special gift. That year Harry decided I should have a moped, so he bought me one.

From the beginning, the bike was very hard to get started. It also needed a little push from someone to get it going. The longer I owned that bike, the harder it was to start. But Harry was a pretty good mechanic, so he just kept working on it whenever something went wrong. We struggled along with it for several weeks, and I did my very best to master riding the thing. Then one night, I got on the bike and Harry started giving me a push. I had it on full throttle, and managed to navigate it about twenty-five feet down the road. Suddenly, the bike lurched back, and I was roaring down the street doing the most spectacular wheelie you've ever seen! I had absolutely no control over the bike, and soon there was a quick jerk and we parted company. The bike went in one direction, and I went flying through the air in the other direction. When I tumbled off the bike, I landed unceremoniously in a heap on the asphalt roadway. My glasses also went flying off as I tumbled over and over. After I finally stopped bouncing, Howdy came off the porch in a rush, and Harry joined him to see if I was seriously injured. When they saw all of the blood they really got excited.

All I could think to say to them was, "Shut it off!" I must have said it over and over, but they just kept asking me if I was all right. I finally shouted,

"Shut it off!" I was very concerned about the gas catching on fire and all of us burning up. Eventually, they got the idea and turned the motor off. When we all calmed down, and I decided nothing was broken, they helped me to my feet, found what was left of my glasses, and we headed for home.

One thing I noticed during the moment of excitement was the way in which Howdy reacted in an emergency. He seemed to snap right out of his dementia-like state, and for that brief period of time, he had a perfectly normal reaction to my accident. That was one thing I continued to be amazed about Howdy's Alzheimer's - how he could, on occasion, act as normal as he did before the illness.

The next day I went to the doctor and he took care of the big gash in my shin. No stitches were needed. But a few days later it became infected, so I had to make another trip to the doctor. Several weeks passed before it finally healed, but I have scar on my shin to this day to remind me of my "great moped disaster."

That misadventure convinced me to take the bike to the dealer to get it fixed. I rode it a few more times before I decided I was getting a little old for that kind of excitement. When we moved back to Ohio, I sold the moped to some kid, which officially ended my second childhood.

CHAPTER 13 – BACK IN OHIO

In the spring of 1987, our trip up to Ohio was pretty uneventful. As usual, when we stopped at the rest areas, I couldn't get over how helpful people were. I never had to ask the attendant to empty out the male rest room so I could go in with Howdy, because any number of men were only too glad to take Howdy in and take care of him.

When we made the trip that year, Howdy was behaving pretty well, so halfway to Ohio, I decided to stop overnight at a motel. We were able to get a good night's rest and Howdy slept all night. After our shower in the morning, we had a good breakfast and were on our way once again. The rest did both of us a lot of good and the second day of the trip went by quickly.

It was always nice to see our home again. In both Ohio and Florida, I'd leave the water, telephone, and electricity on. I decided it cost as much to disconnect and reconnect as it did to pay a minimal bill each month at both locations. Also, once you turned the utilities off, you had to drain the toilets, and get underneath the house to turn the water off. I didn't want to go through all of that. Howdy certainly couldn't do it, so it was up to me to do it all. I had to choose the plan that was the easiest for me, and that was it.

It's funny how simple things Howdy did for himself could be such a relief for me. For example, there were still times when Howdy went into the bathroom all by himself when he had to urinate. Even though, half the time, he'd miss the commode, it didn't matter, just the fact he knew where he was supposed to go –was reward enough for me. I was becoming quite a good cleanup person. I just hoped I wouldn't wear out the washing machine, because I sure gave that thing a workout. When Sears made that model of washer and dryer, they certainly made a winner.

The first few days "back home" weren't always Howdy's best. This time was no exception. But we did have a good day after some that weren't so good. In the morning, Howdy went into the shower stall all by himself. While I was washing him, he tried to push me away and attempted to wash himself. Then later on, while taking his nap, he turned on his side, which was very unusual. I always felt his mind was better when he did things like that.

Suddenly, he started talking more than usual again. I couldn't understand most of it, but once in a while, I picked up a word or two. He said things like, "Did he bring the bottle?" I wondered who he was talking to, and when I looked in on him, he was talking to the TV. "She's here," he said emphatically pointing to me. "You're here," he said again. I wasn't sure if he thought he saw me on the TV, or what.

The next day he wasn't content just sitting again, he seemed to be exploring the whole house, as if he hadn't ever seen it before. I knew that wouldn't last very long, as he went through fazes like that on and off throughout the year. He also kept picking things up and examining them. Then he'd rub his fingers over some of the furniture as if he were checking for dust.

On another day, I took him for a little walk before putting him to bed. I must have worn him out because he went right to sleep that night without a sleeping pill. And he slept all night. When I took him on a walk another time, he was awake half the night as if the walk stimulated him – I just never knew how things would affect him.

For a time, I tried to take a walk by myself early in the morning before Howdy woke up. Each time I made a lap around the block, I'd stop to check on him. At the end of my walk one day, I looked in the room and Howdy was gone. But when I searched for him, he'd only gone as far as the other bedroom. I finally had to stop my walking, because I was afraid Howdy might hurt himself while I was gone, and I'd never have been able to forgive myself.

There were times that summer when I thought Howdy's whole system was turned around. One morning at 4:00 A.M. his squirming awakened me. What a mess! He had a BM. I got him into the bathroom and sat him down, hoping he'd finish in the toilet. Thinking he was done, I stood him up, and he went again - on the floor! Finally, I got him into the shower and cleaned him up. Then I took him into the other room and sat him down while I changed the bed. I started to put him back to bed, but he didn't want to get in. As plain as day he said, "No, it's dirty!" I had to convince him I'd cleaned it up. After I got him tucked in, I put all the bedclothes in the washer, and then I started on the bathroom - scrubbing floors at five in the morning.

Whenever we went through one of those exasperating times, I'd be really depressed, and I'd start feeling sorry for myself. But when I thought about Howdy and what he was going through, it was hard to justify feeling sorry for me.

All the bad times were offset by those special moments that made it all worthwhile. Sometimes he'd wake me up in the morning looking like a five-year-old boy so cute with his cheeks all rosy and a sheepish grin on his face. I just wanted to hug him to death.

One day in July of 1987, Howdy and I were driving home from Marion, a town about twenty miles north of Delaware, when I noticed he was breathing heavily. The closer we got to home the louder it got. So, we went straight to Doctor Gnade's office. He was Howdy's doctor in Delaware and he discovered Howdy had congestive heart failure, so he sent us directly to the hospital.

As soon as I got home that evening I called Mary Jane and told her Howdy was in the hospital again. All it took was a phone call and my loyal helpers came to my aid. Early the next morning Mary Jane and Jess arrived from Pennsylvania and met us at the hospital. Howdy was very excited to see them, and I was very thankful to see them, too. After we cried and hugged, we settled down to look after Howdy.

That hospital visit turned out to be quite eventful. For some reason, Howdy started to talk, and talk, and talk. He just went on and on about so many things.

As one of the nurses was heading out the door, Howdy yelled, "Hey there, what's your name?" He wanted to talk to her, but she was quite busy, so she just kept going with a grin on her face. A short time later, while Howdy was eating dinner, he started singing "Silent Night." He didn't seem to have any trouble remembering any of the words either. Near the end of his caroling he looked at Mary Jane and clearly asked, "Who the hell is she?" Then, all of a sudden, he wanted to kiss me, which was very strange. I couldn't remember the last time he was affectionate like that.

Whenever Howdy had to stay in the hospital, we always took one of his stuffed animals to keep him company. I thought having something familiar from home would soothe him while he was in those strange surroundings. On that particular hospital stay, we brought along a teddy bear. Seeing he was in an affectionate mood, I told him to kiss his bear.

He looked at the bear, and then he looked at me and said, "I'll kiss him, I'll tell him to go to hell!"

A little while later, he decided to be nice to the bear. He picked it up and said, "Hi, buddy."

While Howdy was in the hospital, he had X-rays, blood tests, intravenous medications, oxygen, heart medicine, diuretics, a catheter, Haldol, and Restoril (sleeping pill). The sleeping pills made him sleep so much I was very unhappy with the effect they had on him. I thought about asking the doctors why he needed such a strong sleeping pill, but I decided they knew best. Howdy was in the hospital for four days. We were glad to take him home again.

As always, before we left the hospital, the "Home Care Director" paid us a visit to explain the various options we had for taking care of Howdy. She stressed, as Howdy's condition worsened, we should seriously consider taking advantage of the home care services offered by Grady Hospital and also the county's Home Health Care service. More and more I was beginning to realize the merit of getting help with Howdy. When Mary Jane and Jess were there, we could manage quite well, but once they went back to Pennsylvania, it was becoming increasingly difficult for me to handle Howdy by myself. I thought about it a lot as we drove Howdy home that time.

I was eagerly looking forward to getting back into a routine once more, but first we had to train Howdy to use the toilet again. He just didn't want to sit on the commode. When we tried to make him sit, his legs were like two steel rods that wouldn't bend. Eventually, we figured out he had to go down a long way to reach the toilet seat, so we bought an extension seat for the commode, and he seemed to be more relaxed with that.

After his hospital stay, he seemed to talk much more than usual. Since most of his hospital visits involved some degree of lung congestion, they usually put him on oxygen. It occurred to me the oxygen they gave Howdy in the hospital stimulated him. Every time he was given oxygen, he seemed more alert. I began to wish we could have some oxygen at home for the times when he was really out of it, but I couldn't get the doctor to agree we needed it at home.

One day, shortly after Howdy had come home from the hospital, I put his food in front of him and went into the kitchen to get him something to drink. When I turned around, he was feeding himself. I'd cut spaghetti into small pieces, and he ate it all - without any help. That was a perfect example of one of the things he did after having oxygen. That same day, I noticed when Howdy drank liquids, he didn't cough at all. Prior to being in the hospital, every time he tried to drink liquids, he'd cough.

Two days later, after I'd given him his heart pill, he became very unsteady on his feet. He moved very slowly and was extremely unsure of himself. We had to go someplace, and I had a great deal of difficulty getting him into the car. He just didn't know what to do with his feet, and he kept leaning backwards. He leaned backward as if he didn't want to go forward. It was like he thought there was a big hole in the floor and he was going to fall into it. He also had that far away look in his eyes again.

But for all of his unsteadiness and confusion, he could still react to certain stimulation. John and his family had been away on a trip, and when they arrived home, they came over to see us. The minute Howdy heard John speak, and recognized John's voice, he got a big grin on his face.

Sometime later, Howdy seemed to be laboring with his breathing, so I called Doctor Gnade and explained about Howdy's congestion. Dr. Gnade called in a prescription for Howdy, and because I couldn't leave Howdy to go pick it up, John's wife, Betsy, volunteered to go get it for me.

While I had Dr. Gnade on the phone, I asked him why the heart pill made Howdy so unsteady. He said he didn't think the pill was the problem. But after observing Howdy lose his equilibrium every time he took one of those pills, I was convinced there was a correlation.

One evening, that same week, after putting him to bed, he suddenly called for Rusty (me). When I went in to see what he wanted, he was wide-awake and smiling at me. I hoped his alertness would stay with him for a while. When I responded to his call he said, "Thank you," to me several times. I began to think he might be getting better, even though I knew it just couldn't be, but I kept hoping and praying, nonetheless.

When Mary Jane and Jess left for home, I decided we should begin to utilize the visiting nurses who were available to us. And what a Godsend they turned out to be! There were two agencies, one from the hospital, and the other from the county health department's Home Health Care. We used both of them. I called Home Health Care first, and made an appointment with one of the visiting nurses. A very nice lady from the agency came to the house and interviewed me. She explained all the services that were available, and allowed me to ask a lot of questions. I was told what to expect, and what not to expect. Signing up for home health care turned out to be one of the best decisions I ever made. Those nurses were truly a blessing. Almost all of the nurses who were assigned to us from the hospital and Home Health Care were very efficient at their jobs. When the very first nurse came to visit from Home Health Care, she carefully went over all of Howdy's medicines and explained exactly what each was for and how to administer them to Howdy. Some of the medicines had to be given at the same time each day, which I was not aware of, while some of the others had to be taken with food, or milk, etc. She also explained some of the medicines had to be given to Howdy in the evenings, and some in the mornings. One of the new pills the doctor had prescribed was a water pill, and that turned out to be quite a nightmare.

When we started using the water pill, we both had a big laugh. For one thing, you don't give a water pill to somebody before putting him, or her, to bed. Chances are you may be up all night with them, but guess what? I gave Howdy his first water pill right before he went to bed and it was a disaster. Have you ever changed the bed linens five times in one night? Well, I did and I can tell you it's no fun. But, of course, I had to remind myself it was my own dumb fault.

It was one of the nurses who informed me Howdy had a heart problem. I wasn't aware of any heart problems. She said it was nothing serious, just Howdy's heart was beating too fast. Given how everything excited Howdy, it was no wonder his heart beat faster than what was considered normal for his age.

When Howdy began getting small red marks on his feet, I asked the nurse what I should do for them. She said it was not a serious problem. She recommended I buy some lambs wool and use it as a pad under his feet. As it turned out, I didn't even have to go out and buy some as Howdy's sister had given us a supply they'd used on his mother when she was ill.

From time to time, Howdy would get into one of his, "I'm not going to do this!" moods. I always tried to talk to him and coax him to do what I wanted him to do. Sometimes I was successful, and other times that approach met with no success at all. One evening, at the supper table, he didn't want to eat. I told him he had to eat so he wouldn't get sick. Looking a lot like a bullfrog, he looked me square in the eye and said, "I don't have to do anything but die." I had to laugh because that was one of his favorite sayings through the years.

On another day, out of the blue, he wanted to hug and kiss me. It'd been such a long time since he wanted to do that. I cherished that moment, because I knew it might not happen again for a very long time.

The next time the nurse visited I told her Howdy was beginning to shake occasionally. She told me to keep an eye on him if it happened while he was on his feet, and make sure he didn't fall down. She also told me to watch his feet to see if they were turning blue. If they were, she told me to elevate them. She also wanted me to call her the next time he got the shakes. Since he was more apt to get the shakes while he was sleeping, I decided to keep the phone nearer the bedroom.

All the nurses tried to make things easier for me by giving me pointers about a lot of things. They were also good about telling me if they ran across someone who they thought could help me with Howdy. I remember one time in particular there was a woman who could come and help me, but she would have to stay overnight. That was a problem for me because Mary Jane and Jess came quite often to help with Howdy. I needed the extra bedroom for them, so I had to pass on that particular lady.

In Ohio, our mobile home only had two bedrooms - one bedroom and bath at one end, and the other bedroom and bath at the other end. The living room and kitchen were in the middle of the house. We also had a foldaway bed in the sofa, which gave us some added sleeping space, although eventually the sofa became my bed.

In the month of August, the doctor put Howdy on Augmentin. That had to be one of the biggest pills ever made. No way was Howdy going to swallow that monstrosity of a pill. Why they made pills so large, and hard to swallow, was beyond me, especially when they're mostly for older people. After I explained to the nurse that I couldn't get Howdy to take the Augmentin, she told me to put it in a teaspoon and crush it with another spoon. No matter how hard I tried, it would not crush. So I put it in a plastic bag and hit it with a hammer, and that worked pretty well, except for the outer layer which looked like a piece of colored plastic. Howdy couldn't swallow the shell, so I didn't give it to him. I never did find out if there was anything in that shell that he couldn't get along without, but it didn't seem to make much difference.

That summer seemed to go by very quickly. Before I knew it, we were in the latter part of September, and the cool breezes of autumn were beginning to blow. I knew it was time to think about going back to Florida. Each year at that time it became more difficult to leave our family. With Jess and Mary Jane coming to visit more often, and the family being nearby, there was a lot less stress for me. So leaving my "support team" was going to be especially difficult this time.

CHAPTER 14 – RETURN TO FLORIDA

On some of our trips from Ohio to Florida, we'd drive straight through. But when I thought Howdy was up to another visit with the Bevers in South Carolina we'd stop there on the way. Bonnie and her family lived in a small town called Travelers Rest, and that always seemed like an appropriate name by the time we got there. Usually, we'd stay at their place for a few days, which seemed to lessen the boredom of the trip. That short respite also seemed to have a calming effect on me. I truly looked forward to our visit. They treated us like royalty, and we loved that.

As long as Howdy felt okay, we'd go to the malls and different shops to look around and do some shopping while we were there. During our shopping sprees, we'd have lunch at one of the restaurants, and then head back to the Bever's house.

When it was time to continue our journey to Florida, I'd get out my trusty maps. I always tried to pick the shortest route from South Carolina to Florida, but I also tried different roadways from time to time to break up the monotony. Some of the routes I picked turned out to be time saving, while others were not. By the time we arrived in Florida, because it was usually into October, some of the stores would have Christmas merchandise on display already. That always started me thinking about the holidays and what they now meant to us.

One day, after we'd settled back into our Florida home again, Howdy and I were planning on going shopping and he told me he felt funny wearing shorts unless we were alone. It was so hot in Florida it was almost impossible to not wear shorts. But Howdy was insistent, so we found some very thin pants, and that seemed to satisfy him.

We had a big oak tree in our front yard in Florida. Because we'd seen Christmas items for sale in the stores, Howdy wanted to put Christmas tree lights on the oak tree. Since it was still early in October, I tried to explain it wasn't time yet, but I had a hard time convincing him. When I saw the disappointed look on his face that day, it occurred to me I was telling him a lot more negative things than positive things most of the time. I think it ended up bothering me more than it did him.

I found I had to watch him more closely, even when he was doing everyday things. For example, I gave him his pills with a glass of water one day and only turned my back for a second. In a flash, he put the pills in the water and threw the glass in the rubbish can.

On another day, we took a trip to Lakeland. He didn't seem to do much talking, but it always amazed me what he could understand. I thought he wasn't even paying attention to me. All of a sudden, he wanted to know, "What do we need in Lakeland, and why do we need to go today?"

When we arrived at the shopping center I wanted to visit, the parking lot was pretty full. Even the disabled spots were taken, so we rode around several times and finally found a spot. We parked, and I unhooked his seat belt, went around to his side of the car to let him out, and discovered he'd put the seat belt back on. When he tried to get out, he couldn't figure out why he was stuck. I asked him what the trouble was and he answered, "I'm having trouble with this ribbon."

As we got closer to the holiday season, there were some special challenges because we were living in Florida. Being away from our family during the holidays seemed more difficult with each passing year. But having our very good friends, and Herbert and Sylvia, nearby, took away some of the disappointment. At that point, holidays didn't have much meaning for Howdy, but he did enjoy opening packages and watching other people open theirs. Holidays were just another day to Howdy.

That particular holiday season we did have some excitement, however. I can't remember another incident creating such havoc, and yet giving us one of the funniest moments of our lives. A few weeks before Christmas, I finally decided it was time to put up a tree. I told Howdy I thought we should have a live tree that year. He seemed to like the idea, and when I told him I thought it'd be good to put it out on the front porch, he thought that was a good idea, too. It took a few days, but we finally began our search for the "perfect tree." After quite a bit of searching, we found what we were looking for - the biggest tree we could fit on the front porch.

I liked to put lots of icicles on a Christmas tree; so I bought twenty boxes. After getting the tree in its holder, I had to figure out where on the porch it'd look best, not only to us, but to our neighbors as well. It took a considerable amount of time with the preliminaries, but at last it was time to start trimming. First, I put on the lights, then the ornaments, and last, but not least, my beloved icicles. It took me the better part of three hours just to hang the icicles. I hung them by twos and threes and they were evenly spaced on all of the branches. It was a very tedious job, to say the least. After finishing with the icicles, I started putting the houses, trees, figures, etc. under the tree to simulate a winter scene back home. That was also tedious, but when I finished, it was absolutely beautiful!

As soon as it got dark, on went the tree lights and Howdy and I sat in awe, looking at the tree for quite a while before going into the house to have dinner. Before retiring for the evening, we decided to have another look at our gorgeous tree. While we sat there, several of our neighbors interrupted their evening walks to stop and say how very nice it looked. I was quite proud of the job I did on that tree, so I really enjoyed their "oohs" and "ahhs."

I was exhausted from my strenuous day and slept very soundly that night. I gave Howdy a sleeping pill, so he slept all night, too. Evidently, while we slept, we had quite a windstorm. I don't know exactly how hard the wind blew because we never heard it. That was unusual because the house had a metal roof, and when the wind blew hard, the roof rattled. When we finally got up the next morning, we immediately went out on the front porch to view our wonderful tree. With our first glimpse, we realized we'd had strong winds during the night. I don't think there were more than 100 icicles left on the entire tree! But we had the most spectacularly decorated porch screening in the whole park. The screen on the eastside of the porch was almost a solid sheet of glistening, shimmering icicles! I must have stood there looking at that horrible sight for at least ten minutes – speechless. Howdy never uttered a sound either. After the shock wore off, we started to laugh. When the neighbors saw it they broke out laughing as well.

After the hours of meticulously hanging all of those icicles, I had to spend several more hours cleaning up the mess. Periodically, from that day until 1990, when we sold that house and moved back to Ohio, I'd still find icicles somewhere in the yard.

It was about that time Howdy started having a little more trouble wetting his pants. I don't think it was because he laughed so hard at our icicle fiasco, but I was never really sure. But because it hadn't happened very often up to that point, I didn't particularly worry about it. I never dreamed it'd become a major problem.

I took Howdy shopping at Walmart one day and he kept trying to tell me something, but he was pretty incoherent and I really didn't understand. I kept saying "yes," but he knew I didn't know what he was saying. Suddenly, he got very excited and grabbed my arm. He kept talking, but it still sounded like gibberish to me. He let go of my arm momentarily, but a few seconds later he grabbed it again and was talking like mad. He was rubbing the front of his pants. I thought he was worried about his zipper being open, but that wasn't the problem. "No!" he said, "Look at what she did!" When I looked, he was wet. He'd had an accident. It really wasn't too bad, but I knew there were probably more accidents to come. So we went to the girl at the restrooms, and I asked her if I could go in with him. She sent a boy in to see if anyone was inside. It was vacant, so we went in and I took care of Howdy's little problem. In the Florida heat, it didn't take too long to dry, so Howdy wasn't too uncomfortable until I could get him home.

Howdy had been on water pills (Lasix) for some time by then, and did they ever work! There were times when it seemed like he was never going to stop urinating. With all the traveling we were doing, I decided it was time to look into getting Howdy into protective underpants. I was told there were some pants that snapped up the sides and even had liners. You could get either disposable liners or the washable ones. All I had to do was find out who carried them and stock up. Those "hygienic pants" were a godsend. They were so easy to work with and to wash. We used the disposable ones for traveling and the washable ones at home. Eventually, he adapted to wearing the protective pads and wore them without complaint.

Howdy didn't have an accident every time he had to urinate. I could never figure why some of the times, when he got those bathroom urges, he'd know the correct way to relieve himself, and other times, he didn't have a clue. Urinating wasn't the biggest problem, however, BMs were a much greater problem, but at that particular time they were much more infrequent. Cleaning Howdy up often became a major project. Understandably, he didn't want me to know what he'd done, so he'd try to hide it from me. He'd keep turning away so I couldn't see what had happened. Sometimes he'd slap at my hands when I tried to get his pants off. I'd talk to him in a soothing voice and try to calm him down, and that seemed to help. Eventually, we'd get him cleaned up and his clothes changed, and things would return to normal for a while.

What seemed like a really upsetting problem with Howdy having more incidents of incontinence paled by comparison to the news Herbert shared with us on December 19, 1987. He called that evening and was obviously quite shaken. He said earlier that day Sylvia had been complaining of chest pains after they'd taken a long, brisk walk. Later that evening, as they sat watching TV, Sylvia started to cry and told Herbert she could hardly stand the pain in her chest. He immediately got on the phone and called 911. Since they lived near the hospital, it was only a matter of minutes until the rescue squad arrived. The medics told Herbert Sylvia was having a heart attack. They raced her to the hospital where a helicopter was waiting to transport her to the medical center in Tampa. Sadly, the heart attack was so severe Sylvia died before they could get her onto the helicopter.

What a terrible shock it was to all of us. Poor Herbert was devastated. He immediately got in touch with his three children, and they came down to Florida. They made arrangements to fly Sylvia back home to Zelienople, Pennsylvania for burial. The service for Sylvia took place in the church Herbert and Sylvia had attended in Pennsylvania. All of their children lived in Pennsylvania, and Herbert had a lot of friends up there, so he didn't have to go through the whole process alone. We didn't go because it would've been too much for Howdy. That long trip, at that time of year, would've been too great a strain on him. Herbert assured me he understood, which made me feel better.

Needless to say, it was a very sad holiday season for all of us. All the joy and excited anticipation we were feeling for the coming of Christmas melted away with Sylvia's passing.

December 21, 1987:

History and Physical: He is not doing very well. He has been increasingly confused and incontinent of urine, occasionally of stool. This summer he had a mild CHF. But now he is controlled with the medications that are listed.

Examination: He is totally confused. He is disoriented, time and place and person. Physically otherwise, looks to be in pretty good shape.

Assessment: CHF, OBS.
Plan: Continue exactly as is.

When we visited Dr. Hughes prior to Christmas that year, he simply confirmed what I already knew – Howdy's condition had deteriorated significantly since our last visit in the spring. Knowing Howdy was slowly slipping away only added to the somber mood I felt that winter.

We got through the holiday as best we could under the circumstances. When Herbert returned to Florida, we all tried to console him and share in his grief. We gathered at each other's houses and had meals together, as we had before, but those gatherings were very difficult for Herbert. What can you say to someone who suddenly lost his wife, lover, and life-long companion? We all did our best.

Sometimes months went by without too many incidents, or changes in Howdy's behavior. The months between December and March that year were one of the calmer periods in our lives. But I was constantly on edge anticipating the next incident or radical change in Howdy. Harry was staying with us at that time, and even he seemed to be in a calmer mood that winter. I know he still believed Howdy was putting on an act, but I noticed there seemed to be a little doubt in his voice when we'd discuss it. I kept waiting for Harry to tell me he was finally convinced Howdy had no control over his behavior, but he wasn't ready to concede that yet.

March 23, 1988:

History and Physical: Basically getting along all right. Increasingly confused. We reviewed current medications with his wife.

Physical exam: Shows he is totally confused. Really would not carry on any conversation at all today. Lungs basically clear. Heart sounds are normal.

Assessment: Severe organic brain syndrome.
Plan: I refilled his prescriptions.

I was pleased the doctors always took the time to explain about Howdy's medications. But I still had to find out if they worked the way they were supposed to work. Sometimes they did, and sometimes they didn't.

In early spring that year, I was especially looking forward to getting settled back into our house trailer in Delaware, and being with our family again. With the loss of Sylvia, and Howdy slipping further into Alzheimer's each month, I felt we had to get to our Ohio home the quickest way possible. Therefore, I decided to drive straight through again. We didn't make an overnight stop at a motel, but just stopped when we absolutely had to for food, or coffee, or to go to the restroom. Howdy slept most of the time, and I couldn't wake him, so that helped to make the decision for me. Once again, I was very grateful for the helpful people who gave me a hand with Howdy. And, as always, I didn't even have to ask for help.

PHOTO GALLERY

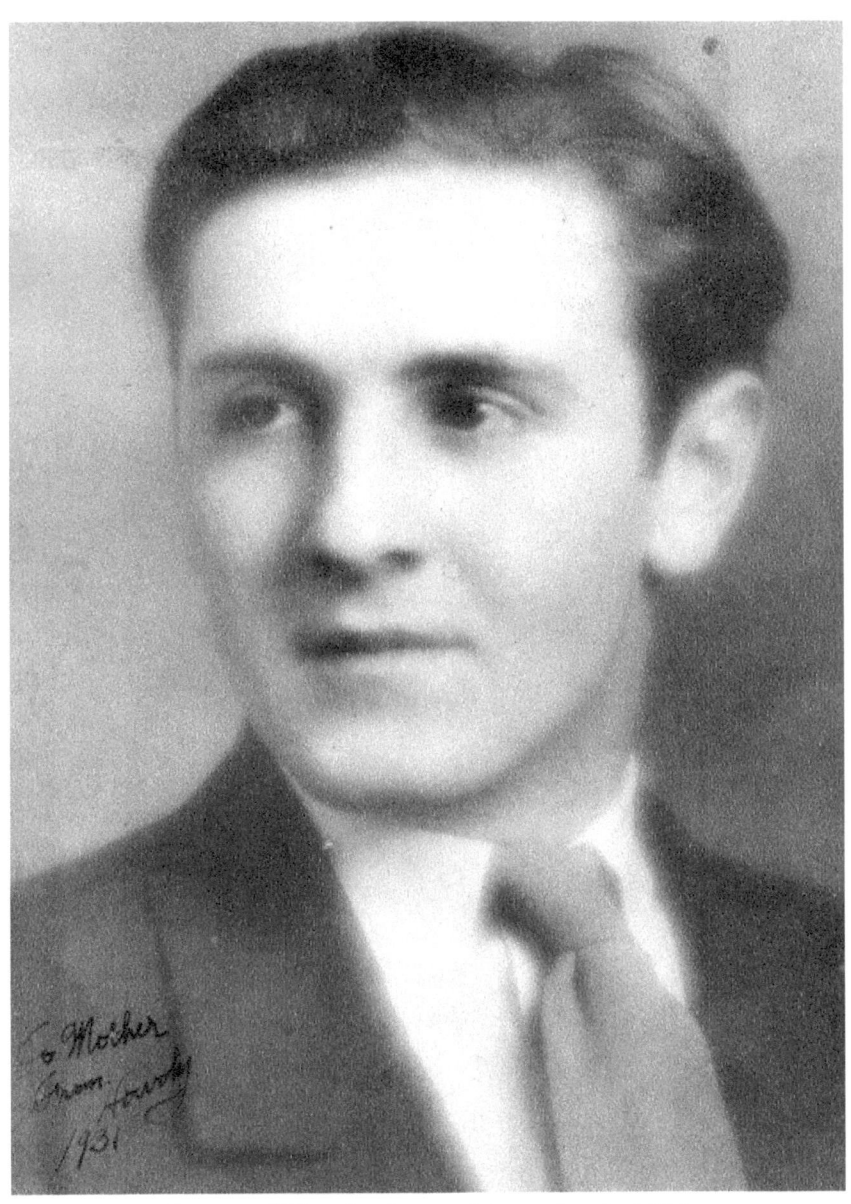

Picture of Howdy given to his mother in 1931

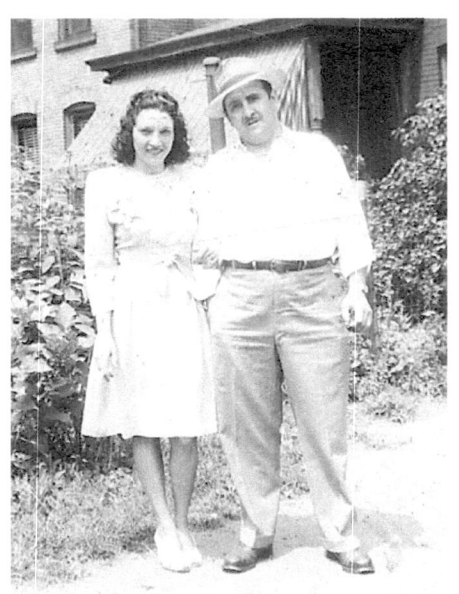

Howdy and Rusty early on

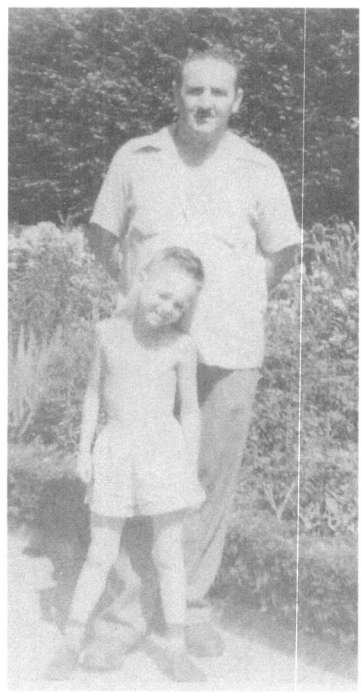

Howdy and John at Niagara Falls in September of 1949

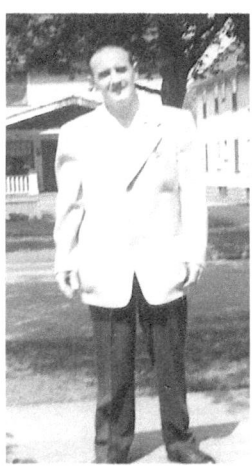

Howdy in front of our house on East 154th Street in Cleveland

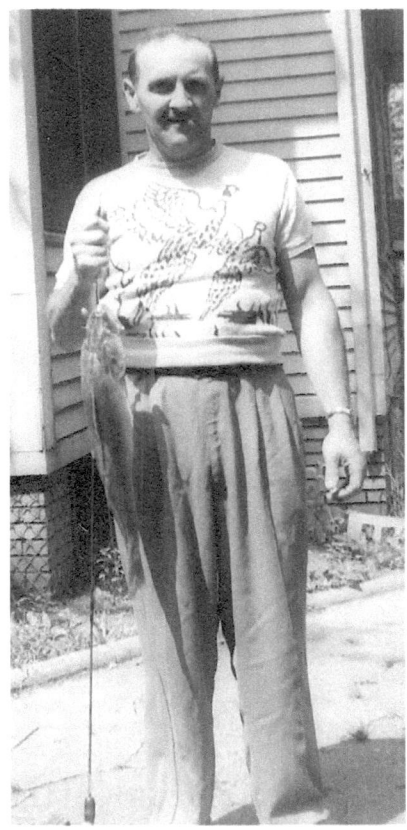

Howdy back from Lake Erie with his catch

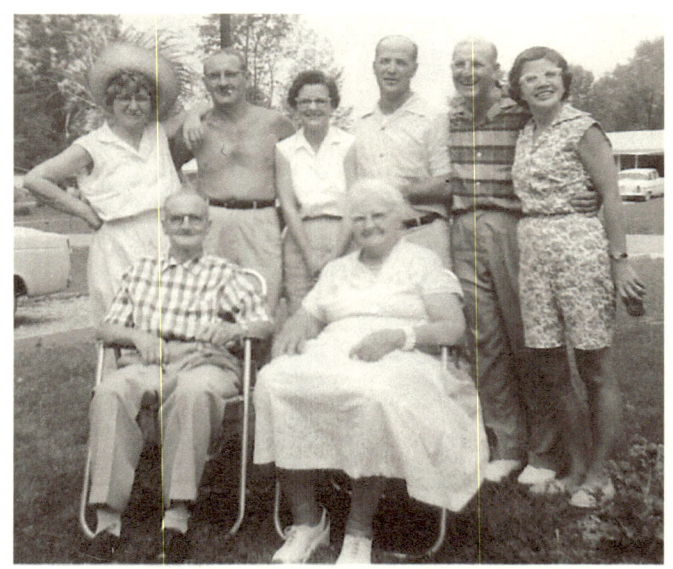

Howdy with his brothers and sisters standing
behind their mother and father

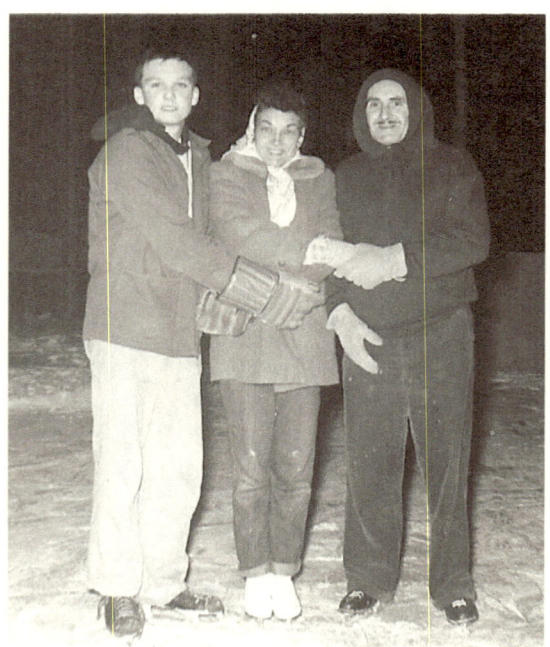

John, Rusty, and Howdy skating on the ice rink in the backyard of their
Brunswick house 1959

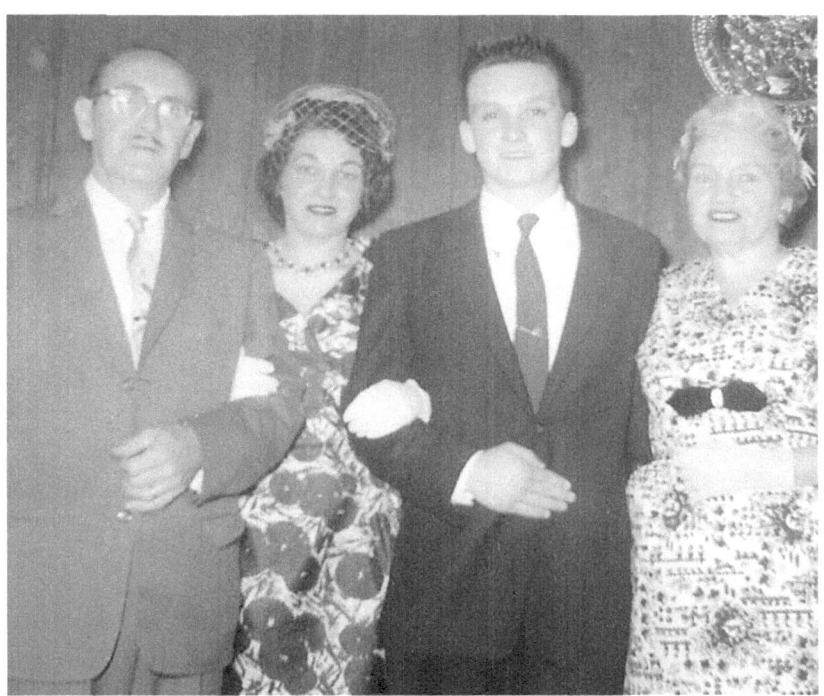

John's high school graduation in May of 1960 with Howdy, Rusty, and Rusty's mother Hilda

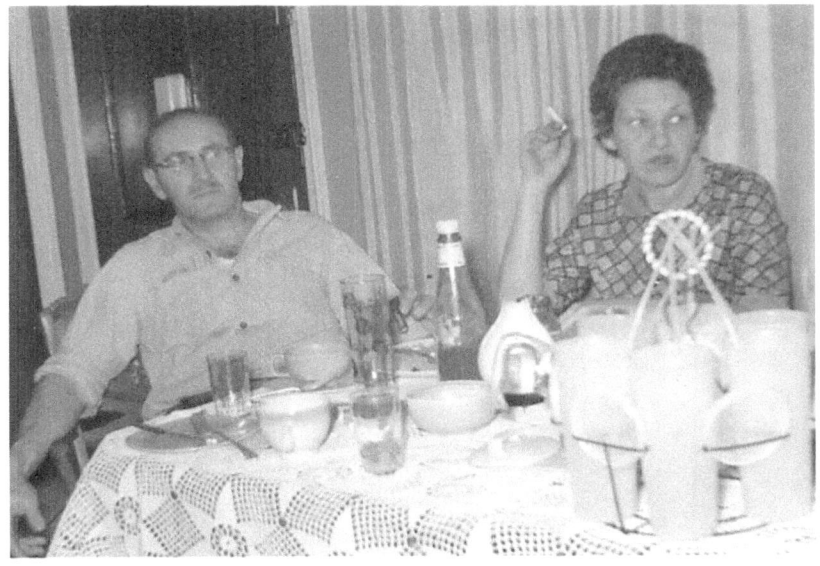

Howdy and Rusty August 1961

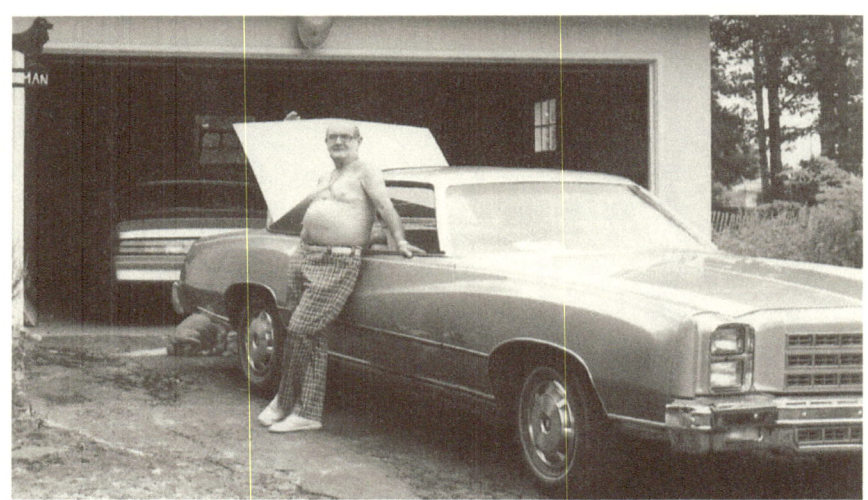

Howdy in front of the Brunswick house

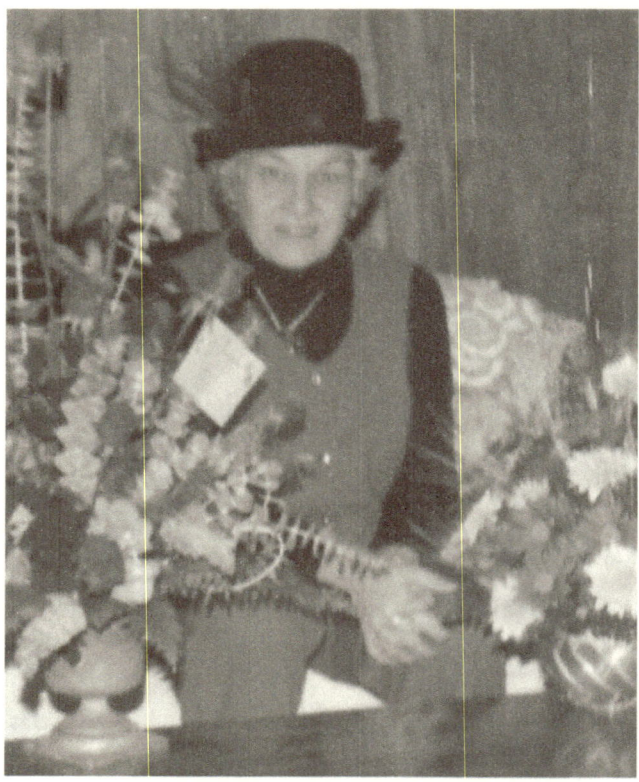

Rusty always loved her hats

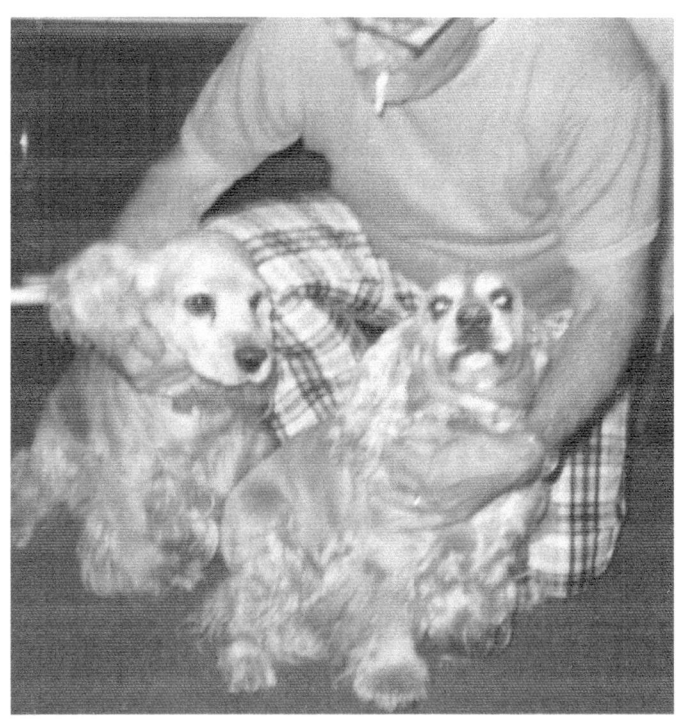

Howdy with Smoky and Misty

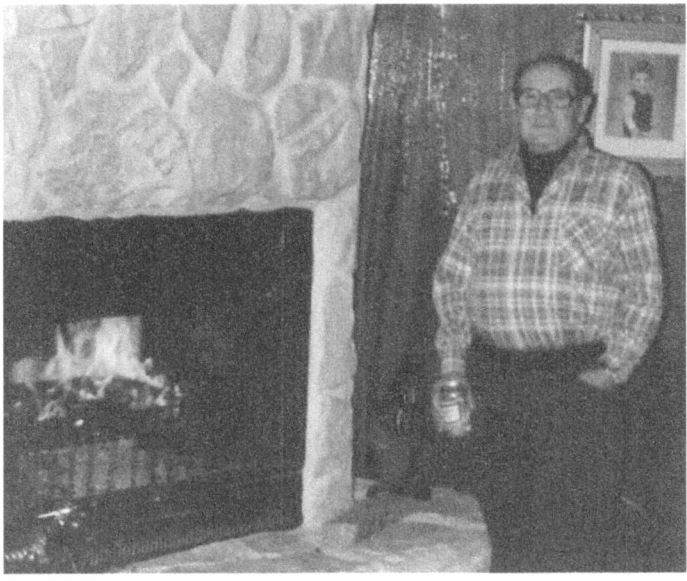

Howdy standing next to the fireplace in the Brunswick house

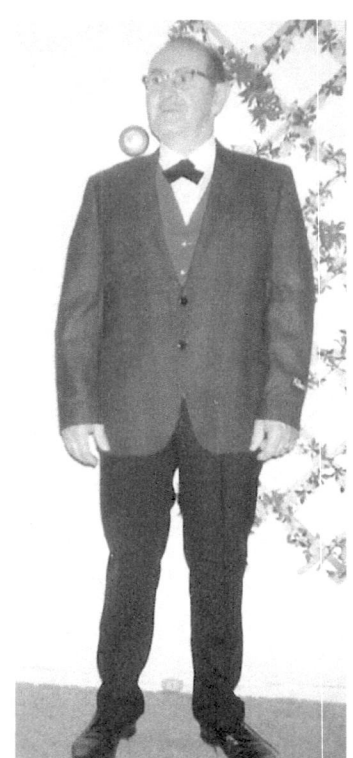

Howdy Christmas 1967

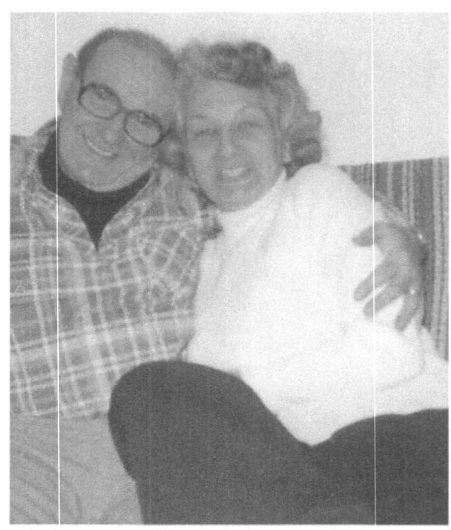

Howdy and Rusty 1978

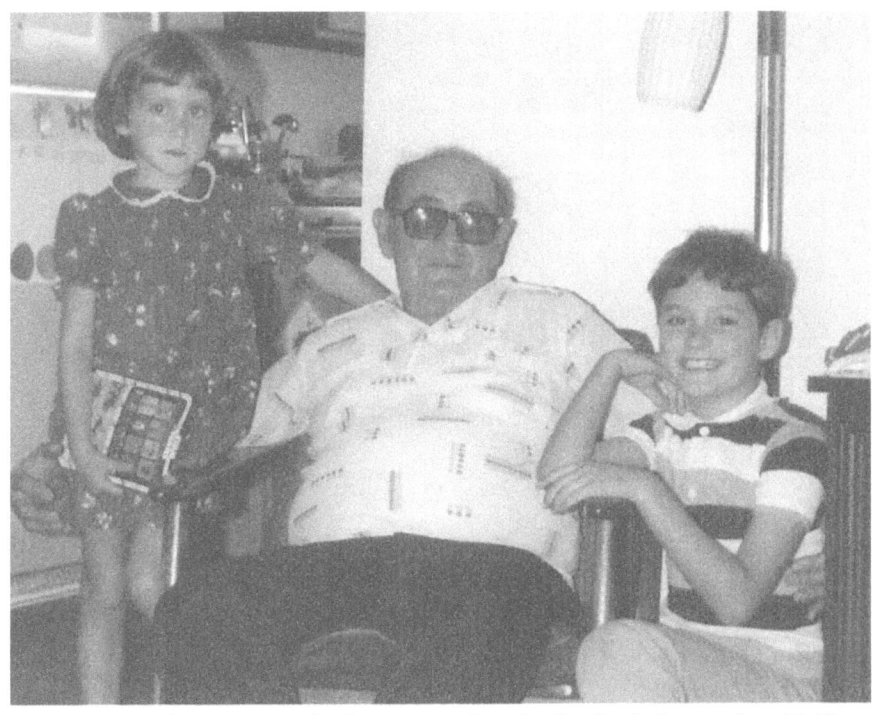

Howdy with Janean and John Howard at the Becker's September 1979

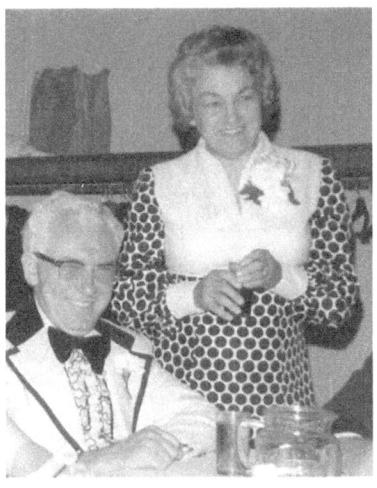

Harry and Rusty at a family wedding

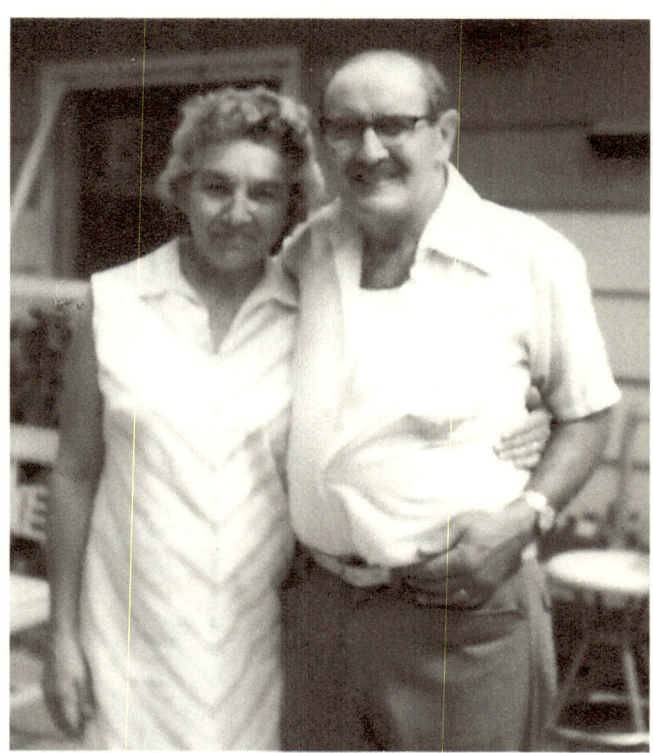

Howdy and Rusty on the patio of our Brunswick home

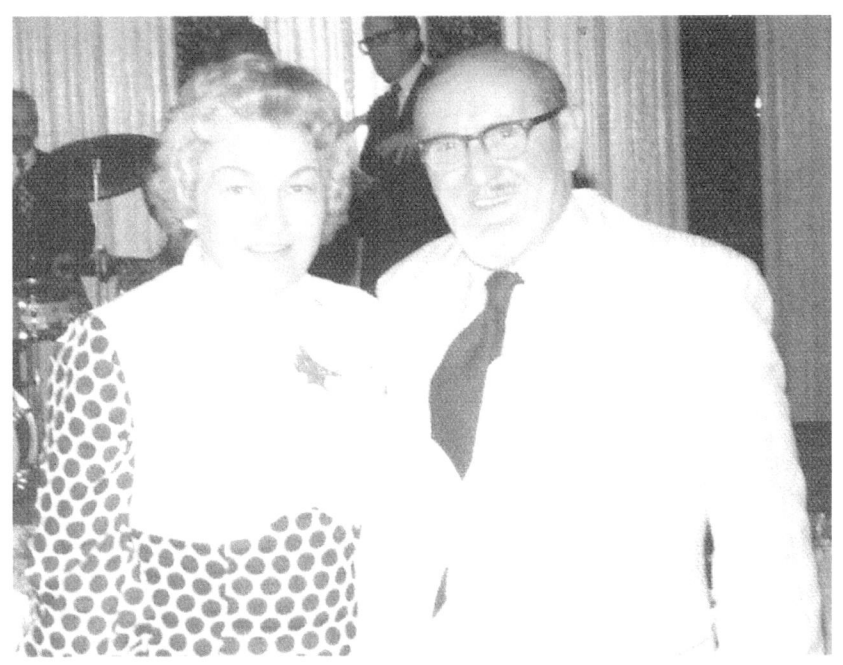

Howdy sporting a goatee and Rusty ready for a night of partying

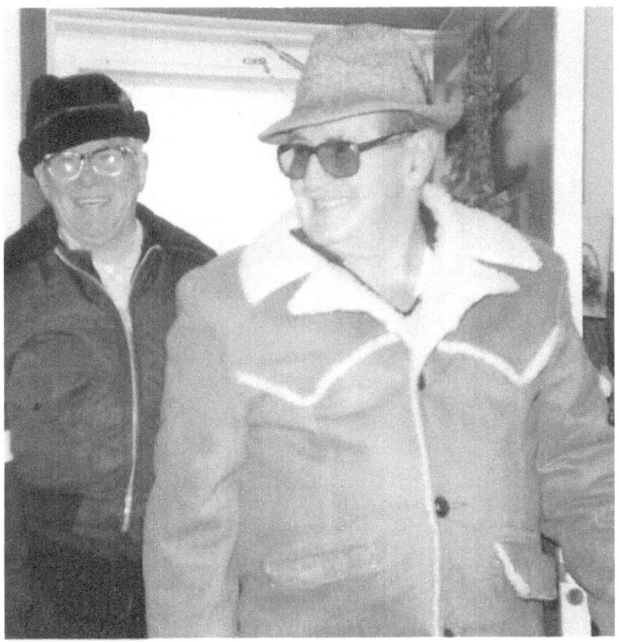

Howdy and Harry visiting the Beckers for Christmas

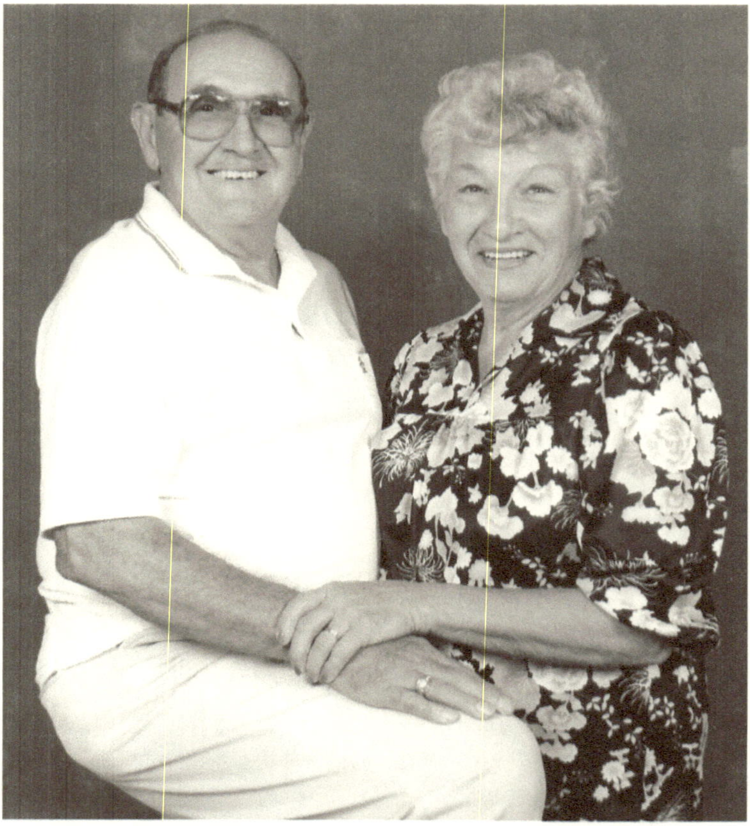

Howdy and Rusty in their blissful retirement

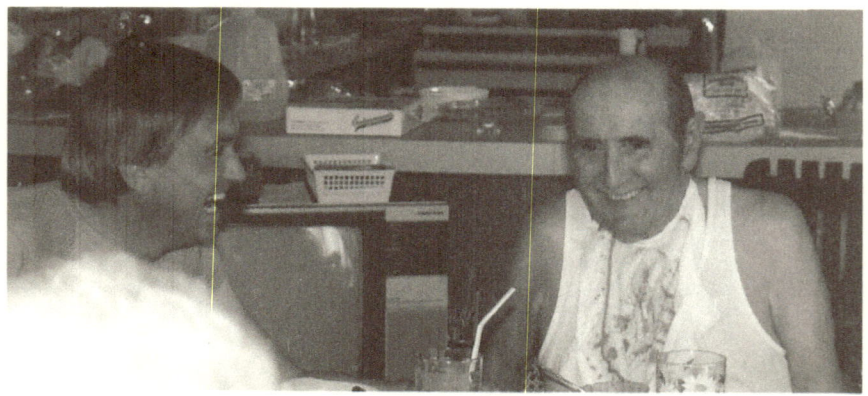

John and Howdy sharing a laugh in June 1987

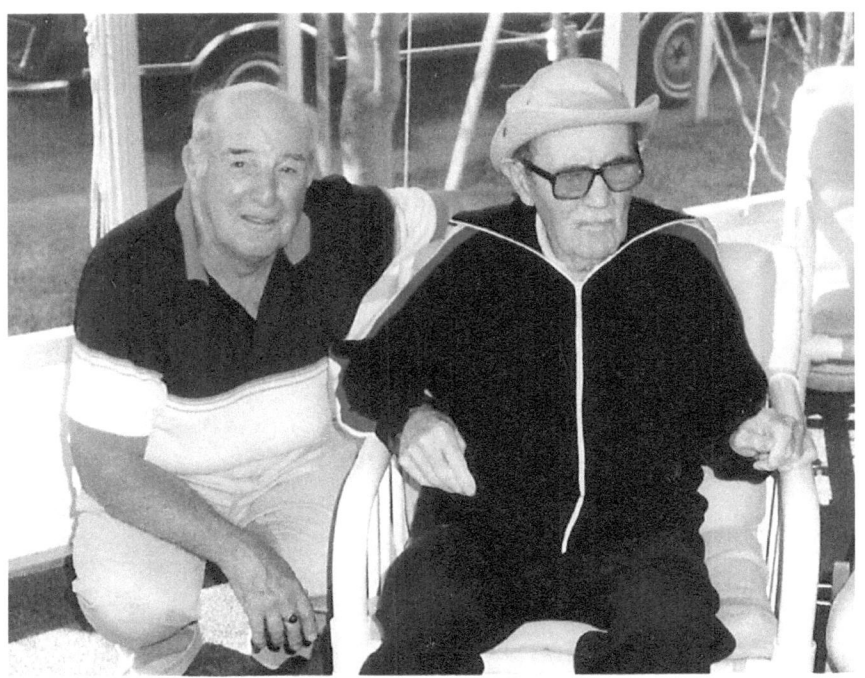

Herb and Howdy March 1989

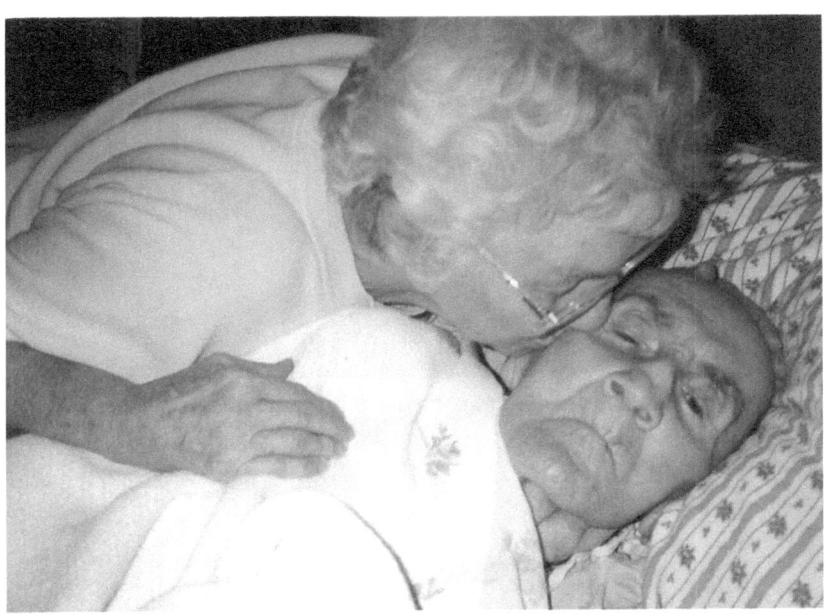

Rusty kissing her beloved Howdy during the final stage of his illness

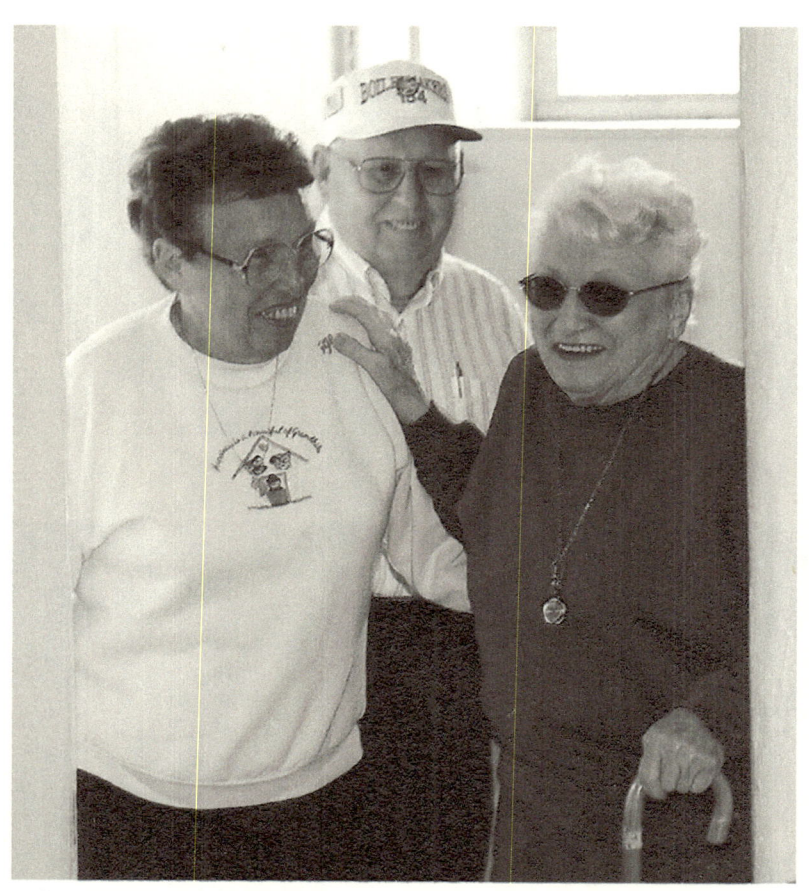

Rusty's surprise 80th birthday party with Mary Jane and Jess October, 2001

CHAPTER 15 – HOME IN OHIO AGAIN

On the trip to Ohio in the spring of 1988, we ran into some of the worse rainstorms I'd ever seen. We always took I-75 north until we got into Cincinnati, and there we jogged over to I-71, which we then followed the rest of the way to Columbus. By the time we reached the outskirts of Cincinnati, it was really pouring. It was raining so hard, and it was so dark, I could hardly see the road. Being as drowsy as I was, I should have pulled over someplace, but I was desperate to get home and I didn't want to stop just two hours away.

Thank God for truckers! There were a lot of times I thought they drove too fast, but not that night. I decided to pull in behind one of the trucks and stick with him. Visibility was terrible, so I followed him right through Cincinnati hoping he was going to Columbus and not up I-75 to Michigan. My eyes were glued to his rear lights, and they were my beacon in the gloomy night. He was really highballing, but I hung with him for about an hour until he got us all the way through Cincinnati. Without him, I would've had to pull off the road. Once we were out of the city, I realized what a miracle it was I had him to get us through that treacherous stretch of highway under the worst possible conditions.

Fortunately, he was going toward Columbus. As soon as I knew we were on I-71 heading in the right direction, I pulled around him. As I went by, I tooted the horn to thank him, but I'm sure he thought I was just another horn-happy nut on the road.

It rained nonstop for seven hours on that trip, mostly a very heavy rain, not just sprinkling. That was an exhausting and nerve-racking ordeal for me, but a good test of my driving ability. Howdy, bless him, was sound asleep the whole time. He missed the most exciting part of the trip. All together, the trip took about 21 hours. We arrived safe and sound in Delaware and that was all that mattered. That time, home really looked like heaven to me.

Under normal circumstances, I would've cleaned the trailer leisurely over the first few weeks we were back in Ohio. But I knew Howdy's oldest sister, Ruth, was going to be flying in for a short visit a couple of weeks after we arrived, and I wanted the house to be spotlessly clean when she got there. I scrubbed, washed, scoured, polished, and waxed until the place looked like a palace. While I labored on the trailer, I had plenty of time to think about Ruth and what a good person she was.

Ruth was the oldest of six children - three girls and three boys. Howdy was the oldest boy, and he and Ruth were quite close. You've heard of people who'd give you the shirt off of their back. Well, Ruth would've given you her shirt, and her last cent, too. She was one of those rare, kindhearted people who always had something good to say about everyone.

Ruth worked most of her life in a bank. There were many years, especially after her father retired, her income was what kept the family going. She never married, and made many sacrifices for the rest of the family. For years, Ruth made a point of trying to visit us a couple times a year, but for whatever reason, it'd been a couple years since Ruth had visited, so we had a lot of catching up to do. Ruth lived with Howdy's second sister, Grace, in Pittsburgh. Grace did the cooking, housekeeping, cleaning, washing, and ironing. Ruth was the breadwinner for the two of them, with the good job she had at the bank. Ruth and Grace got along very well. They were good friends, not just sisters.

Ruth loved going to graduations, so she was very pleased our son, John, not only finished high school, but also went to college. He graduated from Ohio State University three times after receiving his Bachelor's, Master's, and Ph.D. Degrees. Dear Ruth attended all of his graduations. She was so proud of John.

Whenever she visited us, we always tried to take Ruth out to dinner as often as we could, because she really enjoyed dining at nice restaurants. The only problem with taking her out was she worried about the meals costing too much money. Consequently, she often refused to order what she really wanted, and then regretted her decision later on. It didn't matter we kept assuring her money wasn't a problem, she just felt she had to be cost conscious all the time.

The year Howdy's Aunt Pearl died all of the children in the family were remembered in her will. I'm sure she cared for all her nieces and nephews, but her generosity toward the kids was really because of Ruth who always remembered her, and visited her whenever she could. All the kids got $1,000.00. Howdy and I bought our dining room set with his share. Because Ruth loved to travel, and had always wanted to go to Hawaii for vacation, we all told her it was the time to go, while she had the money. But she never did get to Hawaii. Somehow, the money ended up getting used for household expenses.

When Ruth arrived that spring, we went to the airport in Columbus to pick her up. I'd called ahead to get a wheelchair for Howdy and it was waiting right there for us. We didn't have any trouble meeting Ruth at her gate. Ruth's plane was on time, which was good because I didn't want to be at the airport any longer than necessary. After greeting Ruth, we made it back to the car without incident and I breathed a sigh of relief.

We had a very nice visit with Ruth, but she was surprised at how Howdy acted. I don't think she'd ever been around an Alzheimer's patient before (although Howdy's father had some undiagnosed form of dementia years earlier, his symptoms were quite a bit different). And since it'd been a couple of years since she'd last seen Howdy, the change in him must have been a great shock for her. When it was time for her to leave, our son, John took her to the airport, which worked out very well - no stress for me.

After Ruth's visit, life settled back to normal, or at least our version of normal. As you might imagine, it took Howdy a while to get adjusted to being back in our home in Delaware. He seemed to "discover" new things about the trailer all the time. For example, we had three floor length mirrors in the corner of the living room, two on one wall and one on the other. One day Howdy must have thought it was an opening to another room, so he tried to get into it. He had his face touching the mirror and he kept trying to open it up with his hands. I asked him where he was going, and he answered, "In that room." Thank goodness, I didn't have too much trouble convincing him there was no room there, and to get away from the corner.

On our next visit to Dr. Gnade, he said Howdy was doing quite well. In fact, he thought he was doing much better than some of his other Alzheimer patients.

I can't say enough good things about Dr. Gnade, and the staff at his office in Delaware. The women who worked in his office were exceptional. I don't remember being so much at ease in any of the other doctors' offices we visited. I always had the feeling the people in Dr. Gnade's office were truly glad to see us.

One reason I liked Dr. Gnade was I felt he treated Howdy with dignity and respect. In the beginning, when I had so many questions, Dr. Gnade was very honest with me and he'd say to me, "I really don't know why these things are happening, you tell me because you live with him every day". Even the neurologist in Florida couldn't answer some of my questions, but he acted like he didn't want to admit he didn't know. I always had the impression Howdy began getting Alzheimer's at a time when it was something new for most doctors and nurses. They had to learn along with the patients and caregivers.

The first few weeks after we were back in Delaware, things went along fairly smoothly, but Howdy was admitted to Grady Hospital on June 25, 1988 with pneumonia and congestive heart failure. Once again, Mary Jane and Jess came up from Pennsylvania as soon as I called them. While Howdy was in the hospital, Mary Jane and I made sure we got to the hospital by 6:00 A.M. in order to see Doctor Gnade. That was when he made his rounds. He always had more time to talk to us at the hospital then he did when we had an appointment at his office. I always marveled at how patient he was with me given all the questions I'd come up with. I felt as if I could've talked to him about anything. I especially needed his guidance in getting us through the nights. We went through a period of time when every night was an adventure and Dr. Gnade's soothing advice helped me get through those difficult times.

One evening, after Howdy came home from the hospital, he'd been in bed for a couple of hours when, all of a sudden, he yelled, "Do you need some help?" I rushed in and there he was half in and half out of the bed, his feet barely touching the floor. Boy, did he need help! We both got a good laugh over that one. For some reason, whenever someone around him laughed, he'd laugh, too. Getting him back in the bed that particular night was easy – that wasn't always the case, however.

Shortly after that, we went through a couple more hectic days - bad days when everything went wrong. At bedtime one evening, I gave Howdy a sleeping pill, and it happened to be one of those times when it never fazed him. He wasn't falling asleep, but I was afraid to give him another pill. I desperately needed to get some sleep myself, but he had me awake at least once every hour till about four in the morning. At that point, I couldn't stand it anymore. We moved into the living room and settled there for the night. About 9:30 the next morning, I put him back to bed, where he slept for the next several hours. Why that pill took so long to work that night, I'll never know. We had some crazy sleeping times in those days.

One of the nights, when we weren't getting much sleep, I got Howdy into a chair in the living room. I put a small lap-type blanket around his waist and tight around his legs. That kept him from getting out of the chair, but he never gave up trying. Every once in a while, I'd glance over to see how he was doing. At one point, I watched him slowly pulling tiny pieces of the blanket out and rolling them into a ball. It took him two hours, but he did it. He had almost the entire blanket rolled into the neatest ball you ever saw. But he never did make it out of the chair until early in the morning when I finally helped him get up, and then I put him into bed.

Sometimes, the ritual of putting him to bed turned into a good laugh session. Usually, I'd back him up to the bed near the pillows. Then I'd sit him down, grab his feet, and swing them up on the foot of the bed. I did that with him one night and, gadzooks! Suddenly, his head was sideways in the bed, so I raced to the head of the bed. While I was trying to straighten his head, I could feel him trying to put his feet back on the floor. Then I rushed back to the foot of the bed, and his head started to come up again. While I was occupied with getting his head positioned properly, I felt his feet moving. That hilarious scenario went on for quite a while before I finally got smart and put my foot on his legs and then I finally won the battle. I was always exhausted after one of those sessions.

Things went along great as long as Howdy thought something was funny. When he wasn't in a jovial mood, however, it wasn't much fun for me, either. When I look back on it now, I realize Howdy was in a good mood much more often than he was in a bad mood. Before he had Alzheimer's, Howdy was very easy to get along with 95% of the time.

Whenever we got back to Ohio, Harry would visit us quite often. It was, obviously, a lot easier for him to get to Ohio from Pennsylvania than to get all the way down to Florida, and I was always glad to see him. Even though he'd been around Howdy enough he should've known better, Harry still wanted to believe Howdy was faking his illness. But that year, I felt, for the first time, Harry was finally beginning to understand Howdy truly was having a problem. Much later, when Howdy became bedridden, Harry even helped me move Howdy around in the bed. That help was a long time coming, but it was a great relief to me.

Harry had been divorced from his wife for many years, so he could come and go any time he pleased. Because he lived alone, he always enjoyed eating home-cooked meals at our house. I think that was one of the primary reasons he came so often. He usually stayed about four days, but occasionally, he'd stay a week.

Mary Jane and Jess also came fairly often when we were in Ohio. They never made that long trip to Florida. Fortunately, we didn't have nearly as many emergencies in Florida as we had in Ohio, but I never could figure out why that was.

When we were alone again, Howdy and I enjoyed being out on the front porch, even though it wasn't screened in like our porch in Florida. It worked out well for me, because I loved doing yard work, and I could put Howdy in a chair on the porch and he'd stay put. Quite often, I'd stop my gardening and check on Howdy to see if he needed water, or had to use the bathroom.

It was so nice not to have to go inside to check on him, because I'd be sweaty and sometimes muddy from playing in the dirt. Howdy seemed to really enjoy being outdoors as well. He had trouble getting out of his chair on the porch, so I could almost be certain he wouldn't go anyplace while I was puttering in the yard.

At one point that summer, I started riding my bike in the early morning hours for a little exercise before Howdy woke up. When I did, I always locked the door so he couldn't get out and disappear if he woke up while I was gone. Just about every time I went riding he'd still be in bed when I got back. When he started waking earlier, I had to give up the bike riding. Everything was fine while it lasted, but "All good things come to an end - sooner or later."

As we neared the end of the summer of 1988, Howdy still enjoyed going shopping, although he became tired quite easily. I think he liked looking at the different colors and merchandise in the stores. But he never asked me to buy him anything. I know he enjoyed looking at the scenery too, because he'd sometimes point at different things and smile. Occasionally, he'd even laugh out loud if he thought something was funny. Sometimes, when we were in a grocery store, Howdy would pick up an item and put it in the shopping cart. I guessed he was trying to tell me about a product he wanted to try.

Our house was located next to the community mailboxes for our end of the trailer park. As we sat on the porch, around mail delivery time, people would pass by to pick up their mail. Many of them would stop to chat and they always asked about Howdy. He seemed to like the attention.

Howdy seemed to like to eat lunch out on the porch, too. I figured the open air was better for him than sitting inside looking at four walls. Besides, the fresh air seemed to make him sleepy. Most of the time, he did sleep better after a day out in the fresh air.

When the summer ended, and the cool fall air began to make it chilly again, we had to start thinking about leaving for Florida. I can't say I looked forward to the trip as I had in the past, however, because I knew it'd be an arduous journey. We didn't make a stop at Travelers Rest to visit Bonnie and her family that time. I thought it'd be too much for both of us.

CHAPTER 16 – DOCTOR VISITS IN FLORIDA

On our many long trips to Florida, Howdy usually didn't talk very much. The trip in the fall of 1988 was no exception. So it was quite a surprise, as we neared a turn close to home, when he suddenly said, "Turn here!" Then again, when we got to the park entrance, he said, "Turn here," and he continued to correctly identify each turn in the park complex until we arrived at our house. I didn't realize he even knew where we were until he said that. How did he remember precisely how to get to the house?

After we got settled back into our home in Dade City that fall, the weeks that followed were uneventful. Howdy and I went through our daily routine, and his condition didn't change much. For an extended time after our trip, Howdy seemed to be in really good spirits, and I appreciated that. It was nice to be happy for a period of time. Harry came for his annual visit in October, and things were sailing along so well I never thought about taking Howdy to see Dr. Hughes until early in December. Not having to go to the doctor for a while, after we returned to Florida, was quite a treat, but it didn't last forever.

With Sylvia gone, we made a point of seeing Herbert as often as we could. We were pleased we could help out in that way by taking his mind off his loss, for at least a little while. When he felt lonely, he'd come to our house, and Howdy really seemed to enjoy seeing him. We weren't just related - we were good friends. Herbert had a bubbly, upbeat personality, and he got along with everybody. He had a lot of friends in Florida, so he had a lot of people to visit and talk to, which helped him to pass the time. Usually, Sylvia would've had us all over to their house on the holidays, but that year, we invited Herbert to our house. Since this was his first Thanksgiving without Sylvia, we knew it'd be hard on him. As it turned out, we were able to just enjoy each other's company, share lots of good conversation, and we managed to have a great time together.

December 5, 1988:

History and Physical: There is a self-explanatory note in his charts. This summer he was admitted with pneumonia and mild CHF. He's slowly, but surely, getting worse. He's now incontinent of urine. Totally confused. His wife is still taking care of him.

Exam: He's totally confused. He was non-communicative today. His lungs are pretty clear, but he wasn't very helpful in taking deep breaths.

Assessment: OBS.

Plan: Continue as is. We'll try to get some nursing services to help him.

Dr. Hughes suggested we get nursing services to help with Howdy in Dade City just like the services we had in Delaware. But after investigating the availability of home services, it turned out Dade City had very little to offer. We would've had to go to Tampa, and the travel distance made that impractical, so we never did get the kind of help in Florida we had in Ohio. I had to resign myself to the fact, for as long as we stayed in Florida, I'd be Howdy's primary caregiver. I don't think the doctors thought I'd be able to take care of Howdy, especially to the end. If only they would've seen me later, I think they would've been pleasantly surprised. It was about that time I really started to enjoy taking care of Howdy. I think the challenge of giving professional-type care to him motivated me to become the best caregiver possible.

After our trip to the doctor in December, I never dreamt we'd be going there again so soon.

For whatever reason, as we got into December, Howdy seemed to be falling a lot. We were at Herbert's house on Saturday, December 17, sitting outside on the cement patio. Suddenly, before any of us could react, Howdy tried to get up and tripped over a lounge chair. He fell off the patio into the adjacent grassy area and scraped both his shins on the sharp corner of the cement. They looked like raw meat. And they took a long time to heal, because Howdy wouldn't leave anything bandaged. For as bad as it looked, Howdy showed no signs of pain, so we went home and I bandaged his shins. I told him to be sure to leave the bandages alone. Of course, I knew that was a joke because he'd start pulling the bandages off the minute I turned my back.

When it came time to go to bed, I started to help Howdy get undressed when he suddenly cried out and winced in pain when I touched his arm. I figured that would be a good night to give him a sleeping pill, and that allowed both of us to get a good night's sleep.

Howdy slept through the night without an incident, but in the shower the next morning, he yelled whenever I tried to move his arm (of course, these things always happen on a weekend). I decided if the pain got too bad, I'd take him to the emergency room, but as long as I didn't pull on his arm he seemed to be okay. That night he slept all right, but in the morning he began complaining about the pain again. So early Monday morning, I called Dr. Hughes' office, and arranged for the doctor to exam Howdy.

December 19, 1988:

History and Physical: He fell down last week and hurt his left shoulder. He did not complain about it until he seemed to scream with pain last night. Otherwise he wasn't injured.

Physical Exam: He looks about the same, but indeed there is tenderness over his left clavicle.

Assessment: I think he may have a fractured clavicle.

Plan: I am going to X-ray it. He didn't seem to be in a lot of pain. We will let him know the results.

Dr. Hughes was not sure if Howdy had a fracture in his shoulder, so he sent us across the street to the Humana Hospital. At the hospital we saw Dr. Reno, a radiologist, who took X-rays and also examined Howdy. His report:

Left shoulder and left clavicle:

The examination demonstrates no fractures or other acute abnormalities. There is upward subluxation of the humeral head relative to the glenoid fossa and the acromion has become eroded. The inferior surface of the acromion has become concave. This appearance is consistent with changes due to chronic rotator cuff. No acute abnormalities are seen.

Once we were sure there were no fractures in Howdy's shoulder, I just had to make sure I didn't pull on his arm and aggravate the injury so it could heal. For the next few days, Howdy gradually stopped yelling every time I touched his arm, so I knew it was getting better. Each day he complained less and less. Within a couple weeks, he didn't seem to be in any pain at all.

While all that was going on, we went through a period when Howdy began thrashing in his sleep at night. Sometimes it'd be mild, but at other times, it became violent. I was sure it was related to his injuries, but I was cautious about giving him too much medicine, because I didn't want him to become addicted to pain medication. Once we woke up, that was the last sleep for me for the rest of the night. Sometimes, Howdy slept through it, even when he was thrashing violently. But that's when he'd fall out of bed. Getting him back in bed was the hard part, and that's what got me wide-awake.

After several exhausting nights with very little sleep, followed by restless days, I'd have what I called "feel sorry for Ruthie" days. Sobbing uncontrollably became part of the depression down cycle for me even though I knew dwelling on my problems didn't make them go away. I finally had to tell myself there were a lot of people with much worse problems than I had, and I knew that was true. So, concentrating on that thought, I finally stopped sobbing and gradually began to feel better.

Everything, of course, was complicated by the sudden drastic changes in Howdy's behavior. But I always tried to concentrate on how he felt about what was happening to him. What was going on inside his head?

One day, I noticed Howdy seemed to be squinting quite a bit when he looked at the paper. It occurred to me it'd been quite a while since he had a new pair of glasses. I wasn't even sure he could get through an eye exam, but I took the gamble, figuring it'd be now or never.

I scheduled an appointment with our eye doctor, and now I look back on it, we were very lucky he got through it okay. The doctor did have to tell him several times what he wanted him to do. And he was never completely sure Howdy was doing what he told him to do. But he did get through it, and we got his last pair of new glasses after the examination. The eye doctor told me, however, Howdy could never be examined again, so we never tried after that.

It was around the same time I decided to join a support group in Tampa. I attended a few meetings, but I had to take Howdy with me, and eventually that turned into too big of a project, so we just quit going. The meetings were also held at night, and that interfered with Howdy's bedtime given the distance we were from Tampa. Howdy didn't seem to get much enjoyment out of those meetings anyway. For the short time we went to those meetings, however, I felt as if I learned a lot more about Alzheimer's from that group than I ever did from any medical person. For example, I learned most caregivers who go through the Alzheimer's ordeal think they're all alone with the problem. I was amazed at how many people are in the same boat. And I don't know why I thought only men suffered from Alzheimer's. I was quite surprised to find many women are afflicted as well.

As I've pointed out before, not all of the occurrences with Howdy were depressing. We had many humorous experiences and one that sticks in my mind had to do with Howdy's favorite beverage. When Howdy was healthy, I don't think he enjoyed anything more than a cold glass of beer. So, I decided one day since he wasn't allowed to drink alcohol anymore, I'd buy him some non-alcoholic beer. One morning, shortly thereafter, I cut a cantaloupe in half and put it on the table for Howdy's breakfast. I had something I needed to do elsewhere, so I left the room for a minute. When I came back, Howdy had gone to the refrigerator and took out a bottle of beer, opened it up, and filled up the hole in the cantaloupe with beer. I stood in amusement watching him gleefully using his spoon to slurp up all of the beer. Then I asked him if it was good. He had a mischievous grin on his face when he replied, "It was delicious!" I guess that's all that really mattered.

Another time, he got a bottle of real beer out of the refrigerator, and when I tried to take it away from him he slapped at my hand and was a little mad. With a lot of persuasion, I convinced him he really didn't need it. I replaced the beer with a glass of pop, and he seemed perfectly satisfied with that.

On another occasion, while visiting some friends for dinner, Howdy decided to take off his shirt and undershirt. He asked me why it was so hot. I convinced him to put the shirts back on because dinner was ready, and I told him we knew he wanted to look well dressed at the table. That strategy worked, and he obliged without any trouble. Sometimes, he was so cooperative it amazed me.

At dinner that night, he put very little on his plate, and didn't eat it all. I knew he liked everything they cooked, so I was a little baffled by his lack of interest in the food. Finally, it was time for dessert. They served pudding, and he pushed his dinner plate away. Then he pulled his pudding dish closer, laid his napkin down on the table, and proceeded to put three spoons of pudding on his napkin. Our hosts both looked at each other in disbelief.

He began to eat the pudding from the napkin with his spoon as politely as you please. It actually surprised me he didn't try to eat the napkin, too. After he finished eating from the napkin, he started in on what was left in the bowl, and finished it all. I tried to act as if nothing out of the ordinary had happened, but our hosts looked a little startled.

No matter what we did during the day, I knew many nights would be sleepless for me. Therefore, to pass the long, lonely hours, I decided to buy myself an Intellivision game. That turned out to be one of the best investments I ever made. That silly kid's game got me through many of those endless nights. At first, I held out hope Howdy and I could play together, but I soon found out he wasn't the least bit interested. So, on many, many evenings, Howdy would fall asleep watching TV, and I'd while away the hours playing my game. Burgertime was great in the beginning, but when I bought backgammon, and a friend showed me how to play, it became the game I enjoyed the most. Backgammon became my late night companion. I just played against the machine, and loved it - especially when I won.

CHAPTER 17 – MORE STRANGE BEHAVIORS

One morning, Howdy asked me where his tongue was. I told him it was in his mouth, and that seemed to satisfy him. I asked him if he could feel it, and he said, "Yes, I can." He then stuck it out and began licking his lips.

"Why did you ask, did you think it was missing?" I asked him.

"Because I couldn't feel it," he replied. I thought maybe he was losing feeling in his mouth, but he never mentioned it again.

On another morning, I asked him how his knees were (he had a nasty rug burn from falling out of bed so often). He said, "This one's okay," pointing to the left one, "but this one hurts," pointing to the right one. He then asked me if I could put a light on it. I asked him what he thought the light would do. He got a very surprised look on his face and said, "Why, to stop it from hurting - what else?" It was hard to argue with Howdy's logic sometimes.

There were numerous times when he could be very rational and hold an intelligent conversation. I can't tell you how much I loved those times. I always tried to keep the conversation going with more questions and talk for as long as I could.

One evening, he asked me if we had any cookies. I told him, "Sure we've got lots of them in the cookie jar - how about some cookies and milk?"

"I'd enjoy that very much," he answered.

He loved dunking his cookies in milk. It was sloppy, but he enjoyed it, and what was a few minutes cleanup? I did try to keep him over the linoleum while he ate, but the important part was he was happy, and that made me happy, too.

Before we went to bed that night, he came out of the bedroom with the bath brush in his hand and a big grin. "I just brushed my hair and my beard," he announced proudly. I asked him, "Wasn't it pretty rough?" "No!" he answered." Then he asked me, "Is my beard on straight?"

I decided to help him finish getting ready for bed. He asked for the soap, and after rubbing his hands with the bar of soap, he asked me for a piece of newspaper. He then proceeded to wrap the bar of soap in the newspaper. When he finished, he opened up one of our chest of drawers, and neatly put the soap away.

I usually got worried when he dumped the bathroom rubbish can in the commode (which he did quite often). One afternoon, he dumped the rubbish in the commode, including an empty deodorant bottle, paper clips, and lots of other things. I wondered what kept him from flushing it down, but I only found the toilet running a few times after he dumped rubbish in it. So, I decided as long as it didn't get clogged, I'd just remove the rubbish and forget about it.

Once again, that winter, Howdy went through a period of time where he sat still for only few minutes at a time. Every time he got up, I had to get up, too. Part of the routine included stripping off, or adding on clothes. He even added layers of clothing on some beastly hot, humid days. But the temperature seemed to have no bearing on his clothes fetish.

Howdy also liked to put on and take off his shoes and socks. Sometimes he'd be barefoot, or with no shoes and one sock, or two shoes and one sock, or one sock and one shoe on one foot, with the second foot sockless, or any other possible combination. He also seemed to walk a little more stooped each day, and to walk slower and slower. I noticed around that time he started to drag his feet a little, too. There were times when I'd look at him and think he looked so tired.

Some days, I thought he was aging right in front of my eyes, then again, there were days when I thought he looked so young, like a small boy, so cute and childlike, and so kissable. He still seemed to like it when I hugged and kissed him - no more fire and brimstone - just comfortable and reassuring.

One morning, I made Howdy toast and asked him how he liked it. He got a disgusted look on his face and said, "Oh hell!" Then he mumbled a few things I couldn't understand. He became more upset because I didn't know why he said, "Oh hell." Finally, I got it out of him he really wanted to know why there wasn't any cheese on his toast. I tried to explain he never wanted cheese on his toast before, but I'm not sure he understood. Fortunately, we did have some cheese in the fridge, so I was able to make him happy by adding a slice of cheese to his toast.

Later that day, his eyeglasses got misplaced and I hunted and hunted. Whenever he put something where I couldn't find it, I tried to think like him - where would he put that particular item? I finally found the glasses in the bottom dresser drawer, lying right on top. He wasn't trying to hide them - he just wanted to put them away.

Later on, he kept pulling his shirtsleeves up, so I decided to take a look, and sure enough, he had two watches on. The extra watch didn't keep him from asking me for the time every ten minutes, however. Time seemed to be so very important to him.

One day, I decided to clean out the shed (we didn't have a garage, only a covered carport with a storage shed where we kept our washer and dryer and all our lawn and garden supplies). I invited Howdy to come out with me, so I could keep an eye on him. When we got into the shed, he spied his golf clubs. He picked them up, and went into the house. He told me he decided to put his golf clubs in the closet because he didn't want anyone to steal them. He must have left them in the closet a full 10 minutes, before he decided to walk around the house with the bag of clubs on his shoulder. Later, when he wanted to hit golf balls in the house, I drew the line. I convinced him the living room didn't make a very good driving range, so he took the clubs back to the shed.

We no sooner settled that problem, when he spied a picnic cooler on the kitchen counter. He wanted to know what I wanted him to do with it. I said, "Could you please put it in the shed for me?" He said he would, but he probably forgot where the shed was located, so he put it down on the floor in front of the refrigerator. He kept looking at it until I said, "Let's put it in the shed." So we did and he seemed quite happy it was out of the kitchen. Sometimes it helped if we did things together.

A short while thereafter, I began to have a hard time getting him to take a shower. He just didn't want to get into the stall. I didn't know if it was because he had to step up, and then step down, or what. I also had to be careful not to have the water too hot or too cold.

One morning, I got him into the shower okay. He was under the water without using the soap for about a minute, then he turned the water off. I handed him a towel and he had no idea what to do with it. He kept folding it up and he wanted to put it away. I kept giving it back to him, and he refolded it. Then I gave it back to him again. I finally had to dry him, as he couldn't figure out how to dry himself.

When Howdy developed a wheezy cough early in March, I took him back to see Dr. Hughes.

March 8, 1989:
History and Physical: He's been coughing for 24 hrs. A deep wet cough. He's otherwise doing well.

Exam: He looks ok, his respiratory rate isn't increased. Tem. is 99. Ear canals are clear, He did have a lot of moist rales and wheezes bilin. the lung.

Assessment: Wheezy bronchitis.

Plan: Proventil 2 mg elixir 5 cc q.i.d., Ceclor 250 mg suspn. 5 cc t.i.d., we'll see him in 7 days, if he's not improved.

I always worried about Howdy's lungs - long before he began to have respiratory problems. I had a premonition that sooner or later his lungs would be a serious problem for us.

After our doctor's visit, I encouraged him to blow his nose often. Thereafter, I realized that was a mistake. I started finding wet handkerchiefs everywhere. Why he kept washing them I don't know, but I suppose he knew they were dirty and should be cleaned. At least he wasn't putting them back in his pockets when they were wet.

Harry packed up and went back north around the end of March, and that's when I started planning our next trip to Ohio. I was seriously thinking about stopping to visit the Bevers in Travelers Rest, South Carolina, again. But, after much deliberation, I decided to call Bonnie and let her know we wouldn't be stopping. Since Howdy was sleeping quite a bit at that time, I thought we should go straight through to Ohio. Bonnie was disappointed, but she said if that was best for Howdy, then that's what we should do.

We had a good trip. Howdy slept most the time, and was no bother at all. After driving 21 hours, we were tired, so it was a real blessing John's wife, Betsy, had stocked the refrigerator with some staples that lasted us a few days. By the time we had to go off grocery shopping again, we were well rested.

I was very upset to learn one of our neighbors in the trailer park had passed away while we were in Florida. I'd been very fond of her, and even though she'd been diagnosed with cancer before we left, and was not feeling well, it was still a shock to learn of her passing. I guess with all the older people in both the park in Ohio and the one in Florida, that was something I should've been prepared for, but I really never did adjust to that type of news.

Once we got things straightened up in our trailer in Ohio, we had to get reacquainted with other neighbors, and I had to get the yard in shape. Having a beautifully landscaped yard was my pride and joy, so I could hardly wait to get started. Because Howdy continued sleeping so much, I was able to accomplish a lot of the yard work, which included mowing the grass, planting new flowers, and weeding. I also spent quite a bit of time on the phone, calling all of our Home Care helpers to tell them we were back, and they could start their services again. Once I did all those basic duties, we settled into our summer routine and the time passed very quickly.

Because Howdy really wasn't up to traveling much, our family had to come visit us. Mary Jane and Jess were terrific helpers when they came. Jess did odd jobs around the mobile home, and Mary Jane did a lot of cleaning and taking care of Howdy. They both loved to cook, so I hardly ever had to do any cooking. In many ways it was a comfortable, easy summer with lots of good times shared with family and friends.

We made our usual visits to Dr Gnade's office, and I never got over how nice he treated us. We managed to make it through the entire summer without dashing to the hospital, and that added to the relaxed atmosphere.

Before I knew it, it was time to think about packing up to head back to the warm weather of the South. I had no way of knowing at the time, but as it turned out, that would be our last trip to Florida.

In planning for the trip, I wrestled with the decision of whether to drive straight through again, or not. I finally decided stopping in South Carolina at the Bevers would break up the monotony of the trip, plus they really seemed to enjoy our visits, and we hadn't stopped on our way up in the spring. I also figured if we stopped, each leg of the trip would be about ten or twelve hours, and we could get several days rest in between drives. The more I thought about it, the more that plan made good sense, and I told Bonnie ahead of time, that due to Howdy's condition, we wouldn't be able to go to the malls this time. She understood, so when we got to Traveler's Rest, we only visited for a couple of days, spending most of the time at their place talking, and getting a good rest before heading on to Florida. The Bevers begged us to stay longer, but by that point, I wanted to get Howdy back home.

When we arrived in Dade City, we had Herbert to thank for stocking up our refrigerator for us at that end. That kindness made me reflect on all the caring and loving people in our lives. It was so nice to just relax and unpack leisurely when we got home without having to rush to the grocery store right away. It didn't take long for us to get into the swing of things back in Florida.

One day, after we got back from the bank, I ladled out some hot soup for lunch. But Howdy wouldn't eat it, because he said it was too hot. So to distract him, I walked with him around the house for a long time. By the time he was ready to eat, the soup was cold. I offered to reheat it, but he wouldn't let me warm it. As he was eating the soup, he spied the butter and put two huge gobs of it in his soup and ate every bit of it. I told him it wasn't very good like that, but he didn't seem to mind at all.

One of Howdy's favorite pastimes was to hide cookies. I'd find cookies in the dresser drawers, on the front porch, on the bathroom sinks, or stuck in his shoes or slippers. Anywhere you looked you might find cookies, even behind the books on the shelves. I tried to put some bread in the toaster one day, and it just wouldn't go down. It was full of cookies. I never did figure out why he had such a fascination with hiding things.

I always kept lots of pictures of our family and friends out around the house, so Howdy wouldn't forget who they were. He was looking intently at a picture of the family for a long time one day. Suddenly, out of the blue, he yelled, "Where in the hell is John Howard (his grandson)?" I asked him who John Howard was, and sure enough, he pointed at him in one of the pictures.

Howdy especially liked to look at the pictures of his mom and dad and brothers and sisters. I couldn't help wondering what went through his mind when he stared so intently and for so long at those pictures. I always felt uncomfortable when he asked where they were, because whenever I told him any of them were dead, it upset him.

One day it was very hot and Howdy was sitting in the living room chair with nothing on but his underwear. One of his shoes was sitting on the coffee table. I asked him, "Are you going to get dressed today? And very seriously he said, "Of course, in due time." There were times when he didn't want me to help him at all, so I'd wait and if he couldn't finish, then I'd help him. Other times he did it well enough by himself, so I just left him alone.

We went through a period of his sleeping a lot more than he usually did, but those times were always relatively brief. One night that fall he slept more than fourteen hours. Sometimes he could go three nights without a sleeping pill, other times he needed one every night.

CHAPTER 18 – HARRY

I continued to believe the doctors didn't know a great deal about Alzheimer's at the time Howdy had the disease. There was a time when I felt I knew more about what Howdy was going through than they did. In fact, a doctor once told me I did. I didn't know all the medical terminology, but by virtue of personal experience, I knew much more than they did about the everyday problems associated with Alzheimer's. If doctors would spend a few days and nights with their Alzheimer's patients, they'd have a better understanding of the disease. And they'd experience, first hand, the terrible stress that goes with care giving. Now, I'm sure, they know much more, but they didn't then.

I always felt Dr. Gnade, our doctor in Ohio, was much more willing to admit what he didn't know about the disease than the doctors in Florida. Dr. Gnade was so kind and understanding about our problems. He always had time to talk to me and answer any questions I had for him. I can honestly say he was my best friend and confidant during those dark days.

One thing none of the doctors could explain, however, was how Howdy could suddenly remember things from our past even I might've forgotten. For example, while we were watching some dogs on TV, Howdy started to become quite agitated. He started looking around the house as if he were searching for something. Then he asked, "Where are the dogs? (Our dogs had been dead at least 15 years by that time). I asked him, "What dogs?"

"Why, Smokey, of course," he replied.

When I told him Smokey was dead, the look of disbelief on his face was terrible. He just didn't want to believe it. He seemed to be remembering things from long ago, but he couldn't remember something that happened ten minutes earlier. That's what I could never understand. After Howdy decided I was telling him the truth about Smokey, he asked me about our female dog, Misty, and we went through the disbelief again. I think the trauma of that situation was as hard on me as it was on Howdy. We both loved those dogs so very much, and I suppose, subconsciously, we both still missed their companionship, too.

When Harry came to Florida shortly before Thanksgiving, he brought Howdy a new flashlight. It was about twelve inches long and held four large "D" batteries. When we aimed it out into the field behind the trailer, it seemed as if you could see forever. One day, I wanted to use it and Howdy had hidden it. I looked and looked for it, and I finally located it, but it was in pieces. All I could find was the body and two batteries. I never did find the bulb or the front part of it. To this day, we don't know what Howdy did with the rest of the parts. I really hoped they ended up in the rubbish. Harry still asked me about that flashlight the last time I spoke with him.

Speaking about Harry, I feel I should explain his peculiar personality. I've mentioned before he couldn't bring himself to accept the terrible change in Howdy for years after Howdy began suffering from Alzheimer's. For a very long time, whenever Harry visited us, he insisted Howdy was acting and doing all the bizarre things he did on purpose, just to get attention, or just to cause trouble for me. It took years before Harry finally admitted to me he was wrong.

At first, Harry's visits were quite pleasant, and both Howdy and I enjoyed his company. But as Howdy became more affected by the disease, Harry's visits became a source of aggravation and stress. Harry wouldn't be with us a full day sometimes before he'd get into a terrible argument with Howdy, and Howdy would get furious. After one of their quarrels, Howdy began yelling at Harry, and what he was saying was totally incoherent. But after a while, it dawned on me what Howdy had told him, and I'm sure he said, "This is my house and if you don't like it, get the hell out!" There were many times when I thought I should have told Harry not to come, but I loved my brother, too, so I put up with the aggravation.

One day Harry wanted to go to Lakeland, a town about 20 miles away and I asked him to please take Howdy with him. I knew he wasn't going to do it, but I had to ask. When Harry said "No," I asked, "Why not?" I explained that Howdy was very good about riding in the car, and he really loved to ride. I promised him Howdy wouldn't even talk to distract him. I said he didn't even have to get him out of the car. He could leave the seatbelt on him, and he wouldn't be able to figure how to undo it. Also, I mentioned with his I.D. bracelets, Howdy would be identifiable if he did get away from him. But Harry said he was worried somehow Howdy would get away from him and get lost.

"Then, call the police," I said. But no matter what argument I came up with, I couldn't get him to take Howdy along. I'd really hoped I might get a few hours respite from the strain of constantly dealing with Howdy, but Harry wouldn't cooperate. As he was leaving, Harry said another reason why he didn't want to take Howdy along was he might catch cold because he liked to ride with the windows open. I just looked at him and bit my tongue.

At one point, when Harry couldn't accept the bizarre things Howdy did, he began telling me Howdy was doing those terrible things just to be mean. Through the years, I've noticed men seem to have more trouble accepting Alzheimer's than women do. Several times Harry told me to put a pair of shorts on Howdy and he'd take him to the swamps and take his shoes and socks off and let him wade in the water. I think Harry was joking, but I wasn't totally sure. Thereafter, I was afraid to leave Howdy alone with Harry even if I had to go shopping. I just couldn't shake the doubt. Of course, there were times when I simply had to go out, but I could hardly wait to get home, and I always cut short any errands to rush home and make sure Howdy was okay. I finally became so uneasy about leaving Howdy in Harry's care I quit doing it all together. Whenever I wanted to go someplace, Howdy either went with me, or we stayed home.

I will say having Harry stay with us wasn't all bad, because he was quite handy around the house and he did a lot of minor repairs and fixed a lot of mechanical problems for us. At those times, I felt terrible about my feelings toward Harry, but they were there nonetheless.

January 1990

Howdy's condition fluctuated up and down for a long time, but we managed to make it to 1990 – but just barely.

Howdy found a very unique way of celebrating the New Year. Harry and I went out into the yard to fix something, and when we came back into the house Howdy had peeled the skins off all the bananas. We found bananas and peelings all over the place. Confetti would've been a lot easier to deal with. I asked Howdy why he did that, and he simply said, "Someone had to do it."

For the next couple of weeks, Howdy kept making wads of toilet tissue I found lying all over the house. Not used, thank goodness, but just dry wads. As usual, he couldn't give me a good reason why he did that, but I'm sure it made sense to him.

When he finally tired of that diversion, he decided to hide a bag of groceries. I was quite frantic because several of the items were perishable and it was hot. Eventually, I found them in one of the closets.

Shortly into the New Year, I noticed Howdy's feet were becoming discolored. He'd always had trouble with his feet, and from time to time his feet would turn bluish and almost purplish, but I figured I'd better take him in to see Dr. Hughes to have him check it out. Howdy also seemed to be rubbing his one eye quite a bit, and he hadn't had a good BM in a week, so a visit to Dr. Hughes was certainly in order.

January 19, 1990:

History and physical: He hasn't had a good bowel movement in a week. His wife says she can't really palpate anything. He's had some trouble with his eye and his wife would like me to check his right foot.

Exam: He looks fine. I think he's impacted on exam. On his lower foot, he has almost purplish discoloration of the right fifth toe. I can't palpate a pulse and it looks like there is some vascular insufficiency in the foot. He had a little sty on his left eye. It seems manageable. His lungs are clear, and his heart sounds normal.

Assessment: Fecal impaction.

Plan: 10% Sodium sulamyd drops for the eye. We discussed his foot. We'll have the nurses go out and disimpact him at home.

After a short while, the discoloration in Howdy's right toe diminished somewhat, the nurses got Howdy to have normal BMs once again, and his eye cleared up after we applied the eye drops for a few days. Another set of traumas dealt with successfully.

From time to time, Howdy would come up with something quite amusing. I walked into the living room one day and he said, "Watch this!" Then he put his finger in his mouth, got it wet, and hit the palm of his hand with it. "Now, watch this!" he said with a bit more flourish, and he wet his fingertip again, and then he hit the tips of the fingers on his other hand twice each. It was something to watch his face, because he really thought he'd done a neat trick. The big grin on his face showed he was quite pleased with himself and I acted impressed as well. We did have some hilarity in our lives after all. I was grateful he still had a good sense of humor.

A neighbor came to visit the next morning, and I was still in my robe. She thought I might be a little under the weather. I said, "No, I'm waiting for Howdy to get up, so I can give him his shower." While we were still talking, Howdy came down the hall in his under shorts. He paraded into the living room as if he'd been fully clothed. I wish I had a photograph of the shocked look on that lady's face. Howdy wasn't the least bit embarrassed, but I was, for both of us.

We had several small plastic tables on the front porch. They weren't very sturdy, but they were good enough to use as end tables. One morning, I left Howdy alone on the front porch while I did some house cleaning. He decided to use the tables as chairs, because he sat on three of them. When I found them, they were only good for trash. Fortunately, he didn't get hurt in the process. So we lost three tables, so what. I'm amazed at how often I said to myself, "So what," instead of getting mad. I normally have a short fuse, but I'm pleased at how well I handled most of the disasters by that time. In many ways, I was like a whole new person. After most of Howdy's misadventures, I was hard pressed to be mad at him when he had the innocent look on his face of an angelic child. That went a long way toward helping me to keep calm and cool.

Occasionally, he'd hide things like the mail, his watch, and even his glasses. Sometimes, when those items disappeared, he might eventually remember what he did with them, but usually he didn't remember at all. I had to find them, and sometimes I did, and sometimes I didn't.

One evening, we went out to dinner with friends and we all drank coffee, including Howdy. I was starting to believe that caffeine had a bad effect on him, but I let him drink the coffee anyhow. After we got home, at around ten o'clock, he was still wide-awake. I waited until 10:30 hoping he'd become sleepy, but he was still flying high, so I gave him a sleeping pill. He finally went to sleep, but 10 minutes later, he was standing in the hallway sporting a playful grin. The rest of that night, I kept putting him to bed, but I'd look up to see him standing in the hallway grinning like a Cheshire cat. After 5 or 6 attempts, I realized we weren't going to get any sleep that night. Not only was he wide-awake, but he was in one of his talkative moods. He just kept talking, even when I put him in bed, he kept right on talking. He couldn't stop - it was like someone had wound him up. I finally decided it was no use, so I brought him into the living room, put him on a chair, wrapped him in a blanket, and that's where we spent the night.

The next day, I decided to give him an extra half pill before he went to bed. I was getting pretty desperate to get some sleep, and ready to resort to desperate measures. Actually, the doctor thought Howdy needed more medicine, but he didn't see what it did to him. I was adamant I didn't want him sleeping all the time. That night, it took until 4:00 A.M. before he got sleepy, even with the extra half pill. So we trudged off to bed, and he only got up once the rest of the night. Thank God for small miracles! The next day, he slept till 4:00 P.M. At 8:00 P.M., he was back in bed again. I blamed the caffeine for causing that disruption to our lives.

We had a set of wood coasters with cork centers in them. Each coaster had a small brad in it that held a small ball in place which was used to pull the coasters out of their container. Howdy was playing with them one evening when I realized he was chewing on something. I asked him what he was chewing on, but he didn't want to open his mouth to show me. When I finally convinced him to let me look, there was a ball in his mouth. After checking the coasters there was still one brad missing, but I never found it. I still don't know if he swallowed it, or it got lost in the carpeting.

Howdy hardly ever helped himself to food, so when I found him eating a banana one morning I was surprised. There were no peelings anywhere, so I started looking for them, because I didn't want them lying around, especially in the hot Florida weather. I looked and looked and looked, and finally I found them hidden behind some books on a shelf in the living room.

That afternoon, we went shopping at a mall in Lakeland. I decided we needed to use the escalator. Well, what a joke that turned out to be. After about four tries, we finally made it. But all the way up, I kept worrying about Howdy getting caught in the thing. Thereafter, I decided it might be wiser to use the elevator.

If we were in a store someplace, and I took too much time looking at the merchandise and not paying enough attention to Howdy, he'd disappear. It never ceased to amaze me how someone that slow could move so quickly when he wanted to get away from me. It's no wonder those shopping trips wore him out. As soon as we got home after one of our shopping excursions, I'd put him down for a nap. No matter how many times he napped during the course of a day, when he got up, he always made the bed, and very neatly too, bedspread and all.

I watched him examining the dining room furniture quite intently one day, and as he continued his inspection, he kept rubbing his hands over the table and chairs. Then he asked me, "Where did all this cheap furniture come from?" I almost choked, because it was the most expensive furniture we owned.

Howdy really seemed to miss me when I went away. I took him to stay with Herb while I went to the eye doctor one afternoon. But, after I picked him up, he acted funny - very morose and dejected. For the rest of the day, he followed me everywhere I went. In fact, he followed me so closely that when I stopped he ran into me. It became quite obvious he didn't want to let me out of his sight, because he was afraid I'd go off and leave him again. I appreciated he missed me as much as he did, but it got to be a problem with him right on my heels.

Periodically, he'd become very alert again. The next time I had an appointment to see the eye doctor I decided to take Howdy with me. When I was called to go into the exam room, I asked if I could bring Howdy in with me, because I didn't know what he'd do if I left him alone in the waiting room. On the way back to the room, the girl asked how our last name was spelled, and out of the blue, Howdy spoke up and spelled it for her correctly. But the downside of that always seemed to be the better he was mentally, the worse his behavior became. I guess at those times, he understood something was wrong and he couldn't make much sense of it. It must have been unbelievably frustrating for him during those times when he was lucid.

On the way out of the eye doctor's office, there was a bowl full of key rings with advertisements attached to them. They were on my right, and Howdy was on my left. I was positive he never went around me, or reached across me. But, when we got home, he had three of the key rings in his pockets. The only thing I could figure was as I reached to open the door with my right hand, he made a quick grab for them behind my back. A magician would've admired that sleight of hand trick.

Instead of writing letters to our family, I continued to send tape recordings of the events of our lives. Howdy seemed to enjoy holding the mike. When I'd first hand it to him, he'd always say, "Hi! Is anybody there?" Then he'd ask me, "Do I talk in here? (pointing at the mike). Should I tell them how good we are?"

After he gave a health update, I'd ask him what he did yesterday, and he'd reply, "Why, the same thing." He'd then ask how everyone was, and add, "We miss you all. Are we going to see you soon?" I could always get him to add, "Good-bye, I love you all!" Those sessions were always so touching.

We had a cordless phone and I put it on the counter to recharge one day. That evening, Howdy was sitting with a bowl of water in his lap. He was dunking different objects in the water. That seemed to please him, so I let him have his fun. After a great deal of splashing and everything getting wet, I finally got rid of the bowl of water. A short while later I had to make a phone call. When I picked up the phone, a stream of water came pouring out of it. He must have soaked the phone in the water when I wasn't looking. That phone was never quite the same again. When I took it to a repair shop, the repairs would've cost more than the phone was worth, so I decided to just get rid of it and buy a new one.

For several weeks, I got very little sleep because Howdy was up about four o'clock every morning. Sometimes I could go back to sleep, but many times I couldn't. Since I never seemed to make it to bed much before midnight, I'd be exhausted when we got up at 4:00 A.M. Those times gave real meaning to the expression, "short nights."

CHAPTER 19 – MAJOR SEIZURE

Howdy's first major seizure was during the night. The shaking was uncontrollable. I called 911 immediately. But watching him as he thrashed around so violently, without being able to do anything about it, was horrible, and the seizure lasted for about fifteen minutes. By the time the medics arrived it was over, and everything was back to normal. So, of course, they couldn't find anything wrong with Howdy. They stayed for a while to make sure he was all right, and then they left. None of us knew why he had the seizure.

The next day, Howdy seemed fine and didn't appear to have any after effects. But I decided to take him to the doctor anyway.

After the doctor examined Howdy, he came up with this diagnosis:

February 2, 1990:
    History and physical. His condition is the same. He's fairly quiet, he doesn't give his wife much trouble, but he doesn't communicate now at all. His meds are listed. That's up to date and he's taking them faithfully.
    Exam: He looks totally confused, he sits quietly. BP is 100/50. His condition mentally is so bad, I don't think we need to go through a lot of studies; his wife agrees. She doesn't want anything done. If he gets pain and discomfort, she'll return. We'll take a further look at that time. We'll get routine blood work today.
    Assessment: Severe OBS.

No one could give me a good explanation about what happened to Howdy. I asked the doctor if these seizures were going to be an on-going occurrence, but he couldn't tell me. The night Howdy had the seizure he was back to normal before the medics arrived, and all his vital signs were good while they were there. So, how could I expect the doctor to know why Howdy had the seizure when everything was normal by the time he saw him? I was completely in the dark, but I thought of how frustrated the doctor had to be with all his knowledge, because he couldn't explain it either.

Right after the incident with the seizure, Howdy began to tell me how much he missed his family. He seemed to be having recollections from his childhood, years ago, when he and his brothers and sisters were all young. Out of the blue, he'd ask me, "Where are all the kids?" He meant his brothers and sisters. He also asked me where his mother and father were. When I told him they were dead, he got a horrified look on his face, and he didn't want to believe me. It was like telling a child his parents had been killed; it was awful.

During that last winter in Florida, it seemed as if, with each passing month, I had the urge to stay in Ohio more and more. I finally admitted to myself Howdy was only going to get progressively worse. I reasoned being closer to our family would ease some of the tension for me, and would be a better situation for Howdy, too. Even though we had such good friends in Florida, I realized I needed our family close by. I also realized most of Howdy's family, and some of mine, could never make that trip to Florida as often as we might need them. Since I knew we wouldn't be able to visit them very often from that point on, I thought I could make it easier for them to come to us.

Then, when Howdy began having the seizures, I started thinking even more seriously about going back north permanently. Some of the things Howdy did during that time helped to convince me it was the right decision.

Every once in a while after shopping, we'd return to the car and Howdy couldn't remember how to get into it. After several attempts, I'd get smart and walk him away from the car and we'd make another approach. Most of the time, when we did that, he'd get right in. That was another baffling example of Howdy figuring out how to do something one time, but not being able to do the same thing another time.

On one busy day, with many shoppers all around us, and the parking lot crowded with cars, we must have aggravated a lot of people with our double approach routine. But there simply wasn't any other way for me to get Howdy into that car. I tried to explain what Howdy and I were doing to some of the drivers, but they weren't in the mood to listen.

One evening that same week, Howdy frightened our next door neighbor, Aileen Grof, out of her wits. She was in her kitchen cooking, and all of a sudden, Howdy was standing right behind her. She and her husband, Chuck, had their doors unlocked, and Howdy somehow managed to get passed Chuck, who was sitting in front of the TV. Of course, we all laughed about it later, but it scared the hell out of Aileen that night. I think they started locking their doors at night after that.

I found out I couldn't keep asking Howdy questions, because he couldn't keep up with too many at one time. I'd rattle off two or three questions in quick succession, and I'd look at Howdy to see the forlorn look on his face. So, I had to learn to wait and pause between questions.

All of a sudden, he could tell time again. He kept looking at his watch and telling me the correct time. The watch had been missing for some time, but I found it in a cup in the cupboard. Thereafter, Howdy wore his watch and told me what time it was every five minutes.

Fortunately, we had very good neighbors in Florida. They always watched out for Howdy. If he wandered down the street towards the end of the road, they'd turn him around and send him back home again.

One evening, six of us went out for dinner and we were having a marvelous time. When it was time to leave, we headed to the front to pay the bill. I looked for Howdy and realized he wasn't anywhere in sight. It turned out he'd gone back to the table. There he was, walking toward us with the biggest grin on his face, and a fist full of money in his hand. He must have gone back to the table, and picked up all of the tips we'd left on the table. I guess he thought he'd hit the jackpot. One of the men took the money back to the table as we all howled with laughter. Even Howdy thought it was funny.

During another evening with our friends, we were playing cards at our place. I'd already put Howdy to bed, when all of a sudden, one of the ladies, who was facing the hall that led to the bedroom, had a ghastly look on her face. We all turned around to see Howdy coming down the hall without a stitch of clothes on! What a mad dash I made to get him into his pajamas and back to bed. Howdy, of course, was the only one who wasn't embarrassed by his display.

When Harry got ready to leave for home, neither of us realized it'd be his last trip to Florida. The good thing was he could come to Ohio much more often than he could make the long trip to Florida. I also held out hope he'd eventually change his attitude about Howdy, and that would be good for my peace of mind.

The day after Harry left, Howdy got bad again. When anyone left after visiting us, Howdy would always act strangely. Not like in the beginning, when the Alzheimer's first started, but in a completely different way. This time, it was decidedly different, something I couldn't exactly put my finger on. But I knew something was different. I thought after the third day he'd snap out of it, but he just sat in his chair staring into space. I thought that would be the time when my heart would surely break. It was like living in a holy hell – as if the devil himself had come to get me. My mind always seemed to go back to the same question - why? For what purpose were we being submitted to that pain and agony? All I needed was a reason.

After about a week, Howdy finally snapped out of it – once again, there seemed to be no rhyme or reason for it.

Out of the blue, Howdy started something new - talking in his sleep. I could never make out what he was saying, but I figured his mind was working overtime. He just mumbled incoherently.

At the same time he started mumbling in his sleep, he couldn't seem to sit still for more than a few minutes at a time during the day. He'd light someplace for a moment, then he'd be up and moving again. Or maybe I should say he was on the prowl. He was constantly touching everything within reach, trying to read what it said, or figure it out. Nothing made sense to him, or, for that matter, to me, either.

Suddenly, one day he looked at the overstuffed chair in the living room. He got quite close to it, and started to pound the back of it. Then he licked his finger, hit the palm of his hand with it, and gestured like an umpire giving the safe signal. He then made a circle with his third finger and thumb, looked through the hole, and did the same thing with his other hand. As he performed this ritual, I sat in wide-eyed wonder trying to decipher the code, but I never did.

When we'd go shopping on rainy days, I'd leave Howdy in the car while I went into the store. One day, when I came out, he had everything out of the glove compartment, and had also emptied the contents of a miscellaneous box we had in the car. Every single item in that box had been arranged quite neatly all over the front seat.

Howdy also had a habit of taking the cigarette lighter out of its hole, so I finally took it out. Thereafter, I worried if it was safer to take the chance he might put his finger in the hole and get burned, or pull out the hot lighter and burn up the car.

I was very lucky Howdy still enjoyed shopping and riding in the car. At least it gave me a chance to get him out of the house, and it was good therapy for me, too. Sometimes, even if we didn't need anything from the store, I'd take him sightseeing. Howdy seemed to enjoy those rides, and driving was also very relaxing to me. Years later, I still enjoy driving a car for relaxation, and I still miss having Howdy sitting next to me.

CHAPTER 20 – PERMANENTLY BACK IN OHIO

April 1990

In the spring of 1990, I finally made the decision to move back to Ohio permanently. The trips back and forth were becoming much too strenuous, not only on Howdy, but on me, too. I also had to consider the fact we had a much greater support base in Delaware than we had in Dade City. And with each passing month, Howdy was becoming harder and harder for me to handle by myself. So, in April of 1990, we moved back to Ohio for good. There, we'd be closer to our family, and they were such a big help. At that point, I simply couldn't have done it without them.

As I've related earlier, I'd been weighing the pros and cons of moving back to Ohio long before April. But the more I thought about the move, the more the ramifications of the decision became apparent. One of the main things I had to consider was leaving behind our gorgeous mobile home in Dade City. Howdy and I loved that house. Everything about it was wonderful, its location in the park, our delightful neighbors, and the weather in Florida in the winter.

I wished I could've talked it over with Howdy, so I'd have had the comfort of knowing whatever I decided he agreed with my decision. But I just didn't have the option of finding out how he felt about it. Once in a while, I'd ask him if he thought it was a good idea or not. He'd just grin at me, and that was all I could get out of him.

I had become so fond of our friends in Florida that sometimes, in the still of the night, I'd catch myself thinking about them. That was the first time in my life I really had a loving feeling toward my friends. I had friends through the years I really liked and became fond of, but this was different. When I thought of them, I'd get a catch in my throat like I was choked up. When that happened, I became painfully aware I'd never see most of them again, unless they could come to Ohio (some of our friends did, eventually, make it to Ohio for short visits).

I was also keenly aware of Howdy's condition, and I just knew he wouldn't be able to make that trip again. So, I understood I had to decide whether we'd spend the rest of his life in Florida, or move to Ohio, knowing if we did settle in Ohio, we'd never return to Florida again. Either way, there'd be a great deal of pain and heartache accompanying my decision. Then there was dear Herbert, the most thoughtful brother-in-law one could ever imagine. He was Howdy's youngest brother, and a very close friend. Since Sylvia had passed away in December of 1987, we were almost like his immediate family. So, I knew our returning to Ohio would leave him alone, and that thought tugged at my heart, too. But I knew Herbert was one of those people who had no trouble making friends, and he kept his good friends through thick and thin. Several of his friends from Pennsylvania had also moved to Florida after their retirement, so in the end, I decided I didn't have to worry about him. Still, when it came time to actually say "good-bye," I suffered a lot of anguish.

After the big decision, I had a lot of things to sort out, like what to do about the house furnishings, etc. Since our home in Ohio was furnished, and had all the appliances I needed, I felt there weren't too many things I needed to take up north. Harry took my car to the garage, and had a trailer hitch installed before he went home, so I could pull a trailer with some of our things. All of our friends and neighbors encouraged us to have a garage sale, but because so much of my time was spent caring for Howdy, I just couldn't handle the hassle of a sale. Anyway, I'd promised the woman who bought our house I'd leave almost everything.

Once we moved out, the new owners could've moved in with nothing but the clothes on their backs and immediately set up housekeeping. We left most of the furniture, two sets of bed linens for each of the beds, and half of the towels we owned. We also left the curtains and drapes. In the kitchen, we left two sets of flatware, dinnerware, glasses, toaster, mixer, electric can opener, and all kinds of kitchenware. We also left the washer and dryer, and most of what was in the utility shed, including the lawn mower.

With all the worry about selling the house in Florida, and thinking about the move we were going to make, I felt like I wasn't giving Howdy all of my time and attention. Fortunately, he was taking everything in stride, most of the time. Thank goodness, he was on his best behavior while I was concentrating on things that had to be done for the move. Of course, there were some incidents, but none of them were overwhelming.

During that time, there were days when Howdy was actually helpful to me, and then there were days when he wouldn't do anything I asked him to do. On some of his good days, he helped me do some packing. I was pleasantly surprised with how well he adjusted to all of the excitement associated with packing and getting ready to move.

On the day before we were scheduled to leave, Herbert and Walter Schmidt and Walter's son picked up the U-Haul and we all began loading the trailer. Even Howdy pitched in and helped, as much as he could. He'd pick up a small box, or a lightweight item, and carry it out to the U-Haul. I'm thankful Howdy was well enough to pitch in at that time. The move could've ended in disaster, but it didn't. I vividly remember Howdy smiling a lot and that meant he was in a good mood. When he was agitated he'd make some unhappy faces, but there were very few of those.

The only thing broken during the loading process was a two and a half-foot tall wine bottle partially filled with quarters, dimes, nickels, and pennies. There were coins and glass everywhere, and it took a little time to clean up the mess. After we loaded the U-haul, we had a very sad farewell before our helpers went home. Later that evening, many of our neighbors came over to wish us well and to say good-bye.

The trip up to Ohio wasn't too bad considering the emotional trauma involved in saying good-bye and leaving that wonderful house, for the last time. We did stop at about the halfway point to get a night's rest in a motel. It took us two days to make the trip, and believe me, we were sure glad to see Ohio when we finally got there. John was living in our Delaware mobile home when we arrived, because he and his wife had separated. The next day he helped us unload the U haul, and then he returned it to the rental place. Once we unpacked everything, we were ready to begin the next phase of our saga.

Our grandkids came for a visit after we got settled back in the trailer. John Howard had just finished his sophomore year at Wooster College, and was doing quite well in school. Janean had just finished her junior year at Hayes High School and she, too, was a good student. Both John and Janean were great kids. They were both involved in lots of extracurricular activities, while maintaining good grades. Obviously, we were all quite proud of them. Best of all, they were just exceptionally nice kids. But I think Betsy and John had raised them in the right way, so they were good young people.

When they both explained how hard it was for them to get to all their various activities without a car, I started to think of a way I could make their lives a bit easier. I also wanted to reward them for all their hard work at school. So, because I had some extra money after we sold the house in Florida, I decided to buy John and Janean a new car in May of 1990. When I told them what I had in mind, I stressed I couldn't afford to buy them a real expensive car, but a new one as inexpensive as we could find. They agreed to share the car if I bought it for them, and you've never seen two more excited or appreciative kids in your life. I made them promise there wouldn't be any dispute over the car. And it worked out quite well, as they were both very good about sharing. I could never put into words how good it made me feel to be able to do that for those kids. And to this day, they both make a point of telling me how much they appreciated that gift.

It was about that same time, I decided I really needed extra help with Howdy. So, we became even more involved with Senior Services and Grady Hospital Home Care. They were two of the best caregiver organizations in Delaware. I want to say once again what a godsend they were for me. All of the helpers were wonderful, extremely kind, loving, and caring. We never would've made it without them. I can't say enough good things about all of our helpers, from the doctors to the nurses, to the daycare help and the 911 medics. I loved all of them - everyone who made the next three-and-a-half years bearable.

One service came four days a week to give Howdy a bath and change his bed. They came for an hour each day. I could even run to the store if I had to. The other service came four hours on Friday, and I really felt free to do many of the things that, until then, were impossible. Those women were extraordinary in every way. Howdy was always so good for them, and they became very fond of him. They told me he was one of their favorite patients. We were so lucky to have such good caregivers, except one young woman. I can laugh now thinking about her. I don't think she had ever been around anyone in Howdy's condition before. I think Howdy terrified her. When she arrived I told her to give Howdy a bath and change his bed. I had to go to the store for a few things. When I returned, and saw the frightened look on her face, I really felt sorry for her. I think Howdy overwhelmed her. That must have been her first encounter with an Alzheimer's patient. Before she left, I noticed she hadn't done several of the things I'd asked her to do for Howdy. So, I talked to her and found out she couldn't lift Howdy. Then I understood why the bed was a mess, and not too clean. Since I'd returned early, I told her she could go. We only saw that young woman twice. I had no choice but to call the agency and ask them not to send her anymore.

Howdy was becoming more unsteady on his feet with each passing week. Once in a while he'd fall and couldn't get up by himself. I had to learn how to manipulate him to get him back on his feet. I'd sit on the floor facing him with the souls of our feet together. Then I'd take his hands in mine and say, "Okay, let's get up." Sometimes it'd work on the first try, and sometimes it wouldn't. By the time I tried a couple times, I'd be exhausted, and I'd have to rest a few minutes before I could try again. Several times, no matter how hard I tried, I just couldn't make it. At those times, I had no choice but to call 911, and the squad crews always came promptly, and got Howdy on his feet again.

One thing that took me a while to learn was the way to lead Howdy around, not usher him. I'd put out my arms and put his hands on them near my elbows. Walking backwards, I could lead him anywhere without a struggle. But one day, completely out of the blue, he wouldn't let me touch him. That was so frustrating for me because I felt as if he were alienating me, and I didn't want to feel that way about him. It was so hard to look into his eyes and see no expression whatsoever - just a blank look. Was it hate, despair, or was he just lost somewhere in space and time? I couldn't tell. What was going on in his brain to give him such an empty look? The vast nothingness must have been terrible for him to bear. I began to start crying all over again. I thought I'd gotten beyond that. I didn't think there were any tears left to cry.

A full week went by before Howdy finally began to look like his old self again. He even started to smile, like he usually did, and laugh at funny things I did. What a relief it was to feel like we were back to normal again. Those days of radical mood swings were very hard on me, but I couldn't even begin to imagine what it must have been like to be in Howdy's shoes.

Around that time, I wanted to take out his teeth for a cleaning one morning, but he kept biting my finger. After several tries, he finally let me take them out. I could never figure out why some days he'd let me do almost anything to him and other days he didn't want me to touch him.

Then he went through a period of time when he started fighting the sleeping pill. The first night he started doing that, I knew we were in for some bad times. That was a powerful sleeping pill, and if it didn't put him to sleep, then we were in for a terrible night. Sure enough, Howdy got up four times in 20 minutes, after I put him to bed. Finally, I decided to let him sleep in the living room, but he kept getting out of his chair. Eventually, I put him back into bed, and this time he slept for eight or ten hours. At last, I was able to get some much-needed rest.

Those were the times when I was glad I had the books we brought from Florida. I really needed some reading material to help get me through those sleepless nights. I also wished I could just load Howdy into the car and take off for a drive. I still loved to drive and missed not being able to go for long rides with Howdy as a way to relax. Sometimes, I'd reminisce with him about the trips we used to take, and he seemed to enjoy listening to me talk about those memorable trips of yesteryear.

I don't know what I'd have done without our son, John. We hadn't planned on him living with us, but with him being separated from his wife and us having a spare room, it worked out for all of us. Even though he was on the road a lot with his job, he was a big help with Howdy when he was home, and he always seemed to perk Howdy up whenever he'd come in. When John was around, Howdy was in a much happier mood, and he laughed a lot. He thought John was really funny.

The Bevers came up for a three-day visit from South Carolina that summer, and we had a wonderful time. I think Howdy was just as glad to see them as I was. He was also exceptionally well behaved during their visit. He even had a happier-than-normal look about him. The Bevers' daughter, Emily, who was six at the time, was quite interested in helping to take care of Howdy. For one so young, it was surprising how well she did. We let her feed Howdy, and she was really good about feeding him exactly the way we fed him.

The Bevers visit began on Thursday, so with a good weather day scheduled for the following Saturday, we decided to take a trip to the Columbus Zoo. We got to the zoo shortly after it opened, but it was already packed. We rented a wheelchair for Howdy and set off on our ambitious sightseeing tour. It was hard pushing him up the hills (until that day, I couldn't have told you there were any hills at the zoo), but everyone pitched in to take turns, so it wasn't too hard on me. We only stayed a few hours, and, thankfully, Howdy did quite well because he was especially lucid that day. He seemed to really enjoy the animals, but I think he loved the numerous floral displays even more.

The Bevers left for home the next day. Howdy acted like he was mixed up that entire day after they left. He seemed quite agitated and upset because they were no longer there. As the day went on, his behavior got really bad, and he wouldn't cooperate with me at all. Sometimes he'd act like that for several days after someone left following a visit. Making matters worse, Howdy began having a much greater problem with incontinence right at that time, and I figured it had to do with his agitated state.

A few days after the Bevers' visit, Howdy had another fall. Once again, he scraped his knees quite badly. For some reason, his knees and hands and elbows seemed to take the brunt of those falls. We always had bandages in the house, so there was never a problem having the material for wrapping up his wounds. The problem, as usual, was getting Howdy to leave the bandages alone. We'd do pretty well for a few days, usually just long enough for the sores to become covered with scabs. I always held out hope we'd get through the period of healing without incident. But then, one day I discovered Howdy had taken the bandages off, and had managed to pick off all the scabs! What a mess! But my biggest fear was always the danger of infection. Thank goodness, we were pretty lucky in that regard.

Finally, after a few days, Howdy woke up one morning in a pretty good mood. When I got him in the bathroom, and took off his shorts and under shorts, he was fine. But when I tried to put him into the shower stall, he didn't want to get in. So I coaxed and talked to him real nice, and eventually convinced him to go in. That process could take anywhere from five to twenty minutes depending on his mood. Once I got him in the shower, he usually didn't give me any more trouble. Once that morning ritual was completed, our day could begin.

It's amazing how much trouble and stress can be involved in something as simple as going to the bathroom. It wasn't just Howdy having a bowel movement. It was the cleanup after it was over that took so much time, and the stress came from trying to do it quickly, so I could keep an eye on him again. You can't go through Alzheimer's without a large supply of Clorox and Lysol. Medicare should include the cost of those cleaning agents because you can spend a lot of money on them. The way things get flung around and messed up, the germs must run rampant. I can't remember a single day for years I didn't use one or the other of those products. It seemed like I was constantly disinfecting something. That's the reason we had to move from the large bedroom to the smaller one in the trailer. It was simply a matter of convenience. The big bathroom had a large tub and shower, but you had to go up two steps and down to the floor of the tub to get into it. That created such a problem for Howdy, especially when he couldn't figure out which foot to lift up first. The small bath, connected to the smaller bedroom, had only a tiny shower stall with a small step up and then one down. Howdy seemed to handle that one much better. So the move from one end of the trailer to the other was well worth it.

One night, after I had all kinds of trouble getting Howdy to stay in bed, I finally got him bedded down, so I wearily tiptoed into the living room to relax for a few minutes. All of a sudden, he sat straight up in bed and yelled, "Where's the pickles!" I have no idea what brought that on.

I found, over time, Howdy was wearing his glasses less and less. I took the blame for that because, sometimes, I'd get so weary I found myself not as responsive to some of his less urgent needs. Then I'd have a talk with myself, and get back on the ball again. Even though he was no longer able to read at that point, I didn't think that was a good reason to ignore his glasses during the day. There were things he needed to see, so I figured he should still be wearing his glasses.

One of the worst things for a caregiver is to fall into a depression, and to start asking himself/herself a million questions. I guess it's inevitable, but I highly recommend the caregiver avoid being overly critical of their efforts and not question each decision they make. For example, questions like, "What did I do wrong, and am I still doing it wrong?" "Is all this my fault? "Can I do more for him than I'm doing?" You can drive yourself crazy asking questions like that. And you can become totally overwhelmed if you don't constantly tell yourself, "No!" and try to focus on the good care you need to continue giving that person. Keeping your head level is very hard, especially if you have a bad day. And believe me, there will be many bad days, no matter how hard you try to avoid them. So you need to tell yourself, "If I'm having a bad day, what must it be like for him?" That's your only escape, putting him/her first.

Poor, poor Howdy, he stubbed his toe on a chair leg one afternoon, and boy, did he holler. I asked him if he hurt himself, and he said, "Just wait till you get yours!"

I took advantage of the fact I could put Howdy out on the patio, on the lounge chair, and he wouldn't go anywhere. I don't know if he was too scared to get off the chair, or he couldn't figure out how to do it, but that gave me about an hour to be able to do some work inside. The only thing wrong with that plan was my concern he'd wander off if I didn't keep an eye on him. So, I found myself constantly looking out the window to make sure he was still on the chair. I probably would've gone crazy if he'd have been gone when I checked up on him, but he was always there.

Every once in a while, Howdy would still go to the bathroom by himself, and whenever he did, I thought it was great. Unfortunately, I still had to clean him up. Plus, I could never understand how, with all his years of practice, he could miss the bowl so often. During those cleanup times, I learned love is a wonderful pacifier.

Oh, how I loved company! When Mary Jane and Jess came to visit us that summer they brought Harry and our cousin Irene. I hadn't seen Irene for years, and I was delighted she could come for a short stay. What a nice visit we had for a few days. I think Howdy enjoyed the conversation almost as much as I did, because he was grinning from ear to ear most of the time they were there. I even sensed he knew what we were talking about most of the time. He actually talked a little himself, although we couldn't always decipher what he was trying to say. But that didn't matter, because I felt good whenever Howdy made any attempt to enter into the conversation.

The day after they all left, Howdy became quite bad again, his eyes were glassy and he had that blank look again. He was worse than I'd seen him for a long time. I tried sitting on the floor and putting my head in his lap, and he fondled my hair. I really had the feeling he was desperately trying to tell me something. That was one of those times when I found it almost unbearable to be Howdy's caregiver - I just wanted everything to end.

CHAPTER 21 – WHEELCHAIR FIASCO

Howdy continued to go downhill with his balance and his ability to get around on his own as the summer of 1990 wound to a close. He stumbled a lot and weaved back and forth, especially after he first got up on his feet. I figured he was stiff from sitting, and when he got up, he was off balance. After a few seconds, he'd stop reeling and seem to relax a little. Around that same time, I noticed he was beginning to shuffle his feet as he walked and he was walking much slower, too. I also noticed he was becoming quite stooped shouldered.

Whenever we'd go to the airport, I always ordered a wheelchair for Howdy. It was so much easier and quicker to get around with the chair, so I began to think about how handy it'd be to have one of our own. The more I thought about it, the more I was convinced the time had come to buy Howdy a wheelchair.

Once I made the decision to purchase one, I had a few other things to think about. For one thing, because our home was a house trailer, the front door was elevated. Therefore, to get from the house to the car, we had five stairs to negotiate. Getting Howdy down those steps would definitely present a problem, and of course, getting him back up would be even more of a challenge. The obvious answer to that problem was to have a wheelchair ramp installed from the front door to the driveway. John got in touch with a friend of his who owned a construction business, and he designed and built the ramp for us. It was really nice, and worked out very well. The ramp was worth every penny we paid for it.

One of the benefits of having the wheelchair was I could finally take Howdy on long walks around the mobile home complex. I really believe that did wonders for his outlook, as well as mine. He got to see different scenery and other people on those walks. The fresh air seemed to put him in a better mood, and it was as if it rejuvenated him. It always amazed me, after making a difficult decision, how well some of them worked out. After we had the wheelchair for a while, I asked myself why it took me so long to make the decision to buy it.

We really got a lot of use out of that wheelchair. It seemed as if we took it wherever we went, and it made a huge difference. An added benefit of having it was I was getting some much-needed exercise myself. Pushing the wheelchair was much easier for me than trying to hold Howdy up as I walked with him. Therefore, the wheelchair was especially helpful in dealing with my asthma, which had gotten progressively worse as I wrestled with Howdy more and more.

A few weeks after we acquired the wheelchair, however, we had one of our most harrowing/hilarious experiences. I've now told this story many, many times, and it becomes a bit more amusing with each retelling. Because it was becoming harder for me to get Howdy in and out of the car, I decided one day, to take him to the bank and the store in his wheelchair. That turned out to be a **big** mistake on my part. For one thing, having only ever gone to the store from our place by car, I had it in my mind the store was about half a mile away from our trailer. So, on a beautiful late summer day, I was in such a good mood, I decided to take Howdy on a nice, leisurely stroll. As I planned the trip in my mind, I couldn't foresee any problems. I felt quite capable of handling the wheelchair over that relatively short distance, and the first part of the journey went very well. But, about halfway to the store, we got onto a section of sidewalk that was so uneven it caused the wheelchair to start vibrating violently.

I'd packed Howdy into the chair with several cushions and thought that was all I needed to do to ensure a wonderful trip. I also decided to take a rope, and tie it around Howdy's waist and then around the back of the chair. How could I have been so wrong? Once we started bouncing along on that uneven sidewalk, Howdy kept sliding forward, and he couldn't figure out how to push with his feet to get himself back in the seat. So, for the rest of the trip to the store, I had to stop about every twenty feet or so to rearrange him.

As we trudged along, we must have been quite a sight, because some of the passing cars were going real slow and the drivers were watching us. Some of them actually stopped and asked me if we needed any help. Others just watched for a while and then drove off, and some of them waved and honked their horns.

To complicate matters, there were no easy ups and downs at the curbs at that time. Therefore, every time we got to a curb, I had to lower him carefully on one side, and then lift him up the curb on the other side. That required lots of physical exertion on my part, and by the time we arrived at the bank, I was pooped. When we went into the bank, I told the girls how far we'd come. By the way they all smirked at each other, I really think they thought I was joking.

When we completed our transaction at the bank, we had to cross a big intersection to get to the grocery store, and that was no picnic. I must say people were wonderful and so helpful when they saw we were having a bit of trouble. A couple more people offered to give us a lift home. If I knew then what I know now, I'd have gladly taken them up on their offer, but I foolishly declined their help.

After doing a little grocery shopping, we finally headed for home. By then, I wasn't looking forward to that part of the trip. But I'd made the decision to do this, and I was determined to see it through. I'm a little bullheaded, and that time being stubborn almost did me in.

The trip back turned into a nightmare. By the time we started for home, I was very tired, and Howdy wasn't comfortable at all. He was slipping forward and downward in the chair even more often. It was becoming harder for me to get him back in the chair because I was almost exhausted. It also seemed as if he weighed more each time I tried to readjust him.

Regardless of the difficulties, I continued pushing ahead. When we were near the end of the rough section of pavement, I realized Howdy had slipped almost completely out of the chair. When I looked up, I realized we were near a gas station, and there was a man at one of the pumps. I pushed the chair toward him, and asked if he could help me lift Howdy back into the chair. By that time, Howdy was more out of the chair than in it, and dangerously close to tumbling onto the sidewalk. The man was very helpful, and even volunteered to give us a ride the rest of the way home. But, again, I declined as we were now past the rough section of sidewalk, and I figured the rest of the journey would be easy.

After the man at the gas station helped me reposition Howdy in the chair, I was more determined than ever to make the rest of the trip with me pushing Howdy the whole way. We were back to having level sidewalks again, and not too many curbs to go up and down the rest of trip.

Howdy wasn't jostled around too much from that point on, and the remainder of the journey turned out to be fairly pleasant. It still took about twenty minutes to navigate from the gas station to within sight of our house. We were both overjoyed to see it! And I was finally able to relax a little bit. Even Howdy seemed to enjoy the last part of the trip more than the rest of it. I believe we both breathed a big sigh of relief when we saw that little trailer of ours. It truly was "Home Sweet Home!" After our strenuous ordeal, I was ready for a long nap – and boy did I ever sleep. Later, I drove to the bank and back to our home, while I checked the mileage on my odometer and I discovered it was a full **three mile** roundtrip – no wonder I was so exhausted. I'm happy to say I never attempted anything quite so foolish again.

As the weeks and months went by, it became quite apparent we had so much more help in Ohio then we had in Florida. Not just people helping, but truly caring people - people who, obviously, had a lot of love in them. There could be no finer example of loving, caring people than my sister, Mary Jane, and her husband, Jess. They lived about four hours away from us in Pennsylvania, but they thought nothing at all of making that trip every time we needed them. I just had to call, and the next day they'd be there.

Whenever Jess came in the door he'd always say, "I came to help my fishing buddy." Years before that, when we lived in Cleveland, Howdy and Jess spent many hours out on Lake Erie fishing. I had a lot of fond memories of the times when Mary Jane and Jess would visit and the men would go out in a boat and fish all night. And when he became old enough, our son, John, went along with them. He loved being out with the men; being a "fisherman" was a big deal for him. Somehow, I never worried about them being out on those unpredictable Lake Erie waters at night, even when they were gone for long periods of time.

John still talks about the fish they caught, and how he remembers getting back home at breakfast time after some of those fishing excursions. After the men cleaned the fish, Mary Jane and I would fry up the best tasting fish breakfast you can imagine. We still savor those tasty memories to this day.

Whenever Jess and Mary Jane came, we got to do a lot of things we never would've done without them. Of course, having the wheelchair helped a great deal. One of our favorite activities was to put Howdy in the car and take off on a shopping spree. We always went to a restaurant during our trip, and Howdy seemed to enjoy those outings as much as the rest of us. Eventually, however, it got to the point even the three of us couldn't get Howdy in and out of the car without an exhausting struggle. I think he was afraid of falling, so he'd straighten his legs so stiffly we couldn't bend them – either to get him into the car, or out of it.

Sometimes, when I thought Howdy was doing quite well, something would happen, and I'd be jolted back to reality. One recurring incident was especially disturbing. I remember waking up in the middle of the night to a terrible rasping sound coming from Howdy. He'd be having great difficulty breathing. I'd jump out of bed and rush to the phone to call the rescue squad. Within minutes they'd arrive. After examining Howdy and telling me his temperature was 102 degrees, I knew he had congestive heart failure again.

The squad would take him to the hospital, and I'd follow in my car. I don't know what we did before 911.

As always, the next day Mary Jane and Jess would come back again. Mary Jane and I would get into a routine. We always arranged to get to the hospital by 6:00 or 6:30 A.M. That gave us time to bathe Howdy, brush his teeth, shave him, comb his hair and do anything else that needed done. Then we'd patiently wait for the doctor to make his rounds, so we could have a talk with him. That was the best time to talk to Doctor Gnade. He came very early, and we always had loads of questions for him. He never gave us the brush off, and he was always kind and helpful. I really felt close to him at those sessions. I always appreciated he took the time to listen to me. He was always honest with me, and that made a bond between us. Even the two doctors who put a tube in Howdy's stomach in Ohio were very nice and caring. Years later, I had to visit one of the doctors who put the tube in Howdy's stomach, and he still remembered Howdy.

During that period of time, Doctor Gnade began stressing more frequently it was time to put Howdy in a nursing home. It seemed as if after each hospital stay Howdy's ability to get around on his own decreased, and his ability to communicate also declined. So, I could understand why Dr. Gnade felt it was becoming more and more difficult for me to handle Howdy by myself at home. That was the one major disagreement we had. I always told him, "No, I can't do that." We'd discuss the situation, but he never pressured me about my decision.

Even though I couldn't put Howdy into a home, I realize each family's circumstances are different. If a family has no other option, I don't believe people should feel guilty about making the decision to put someone into a nursing home. Fortunately, I was retired, eleven years younger than Howdy, in fairly good health, and had some of the best help you could imagine. There was no question Delaware, Ohio was the best place for us during that time.

CHAPTER 22 – MORE HELP

One of the best things about being back in Ohio year round was being able to spend more time with our family. Janean was in her senior year at Delaware Hayes High School, and into all kinds of activities. It was so nice to be right there and see her all dressed up when she was elected to the Homecoming court during the football season. But it was especially nice to spend the holidays with our family. When Thanksgiving came that year, the kids came for dinner and we all agreed we had a lot to be thankful for. It was truly a Happy Thanksgiving.

A few weeks later, John Howard came home early from college, and he made a special point of dropping by and filling us in on how his third year of college was going. He was majoring in English and history and singing in a campus rock band. It sounded like he really enjoyed school, and was doing very well, both academically and socially. Because he and Janean were so busy all the time, we loved the extra time they shared with us that year.

Janean was also in a talent show at school that year and she sang a Tracey Chapman song acappella. She did a beautiful job and received a rousing ovation from the audience. We were very proud of her!

A couple times, while we were in Florida, John, Betsy, and the kids came down to spend the Christmas holiday with us. But most years, we didn't get to see them during the holidays. That made Christmas 1990 very memorable. It was nice family and friends could drop in whenever they wanted to see us without making that long trip to Florida. Everyone seemed to be very happy, and we didn't even have to worry about mailing packages to each other. We just got together and exchanged gifts. What a joy it was to be surrounded by loved ones at that special time of year!

Another good thing about being in Ohio year round was having our wonderful caregivers working with us throughout the entire year. The longer we were in Ohio, the more I was sure I'd made the right decision to move back permanently.

We were fortunate to have the same women back every year. We became quite fond of each other, and the bond we established got stronger each time they came. And just having the peace of mind of knowing they were right there whenever I needed them was a huge relief.

Even shopping was easier in Delaware because we were closer to the stores than we were in Dade City. In Florida, it seemed as if a trip to the store was a major undertaking, but in Delaware, we could be at most stores we needed to visit in a couple minutes. Unless we were looking to buy something major, we could give our business to Delaware people, which I preferred doing. I'm a great believer in buying in your hometown and helping hometown merchants. For major items, we could always drive into Columbus. Since I loved to drive, and Howdy still seemed to enjoy riding in the car most of the time, we were able to travel to the big city without too many problems.

January 1991

At the beginning of 1991, Howdy was still able to move around and even help himself to a certain extent. There were some days when he'd eat quite well, and there were days when I had to coax him to eat. It was just a matter of my recognizing a particular day as one in which he'd need my help more than another day. Howdy always wanted to do things for himself. Unfortunately, his body was willing, but his mind wouldn't always cooperate.

Thank goodness, Howdy's appetite was still good, and I enjoyed cooking the things he liked to eat. I always wondered if, at some point, he'd forget the tastes he loved so much, but that never seemed to be a problem. For example, he loved pancakes, so one day I made him a big pancake breakfast. He began eating normally, and then all of a sudden, he couldn't figure out how to hold the fork. Naturally, when he held the fork upside down, nothing would stay on it. That made him very angry. So, I had to talk to him to sooth him, and convince him everything was all right. I'd become extremely diplomatic by that point, and I seemed to be using my diplomatic skills more and more often. I could usually calm him down most of the time, and he'd become peaceful once again.

It amazed me how many people in the medical profession in Delaware, Ohio knew who we were. Whenever our names were mentioned in the presence of health professionals they immediately knew Howdy had Alzheimer's, and I was taking care of him at home. That seemed especially true on our many quick trips to the emergency room at Grady Hospital.

Ohio Wesleyan University, in Delaware, had a course of study for nurses at the time Howdy and I were going through the trauma of Alzheimer's. Part of the program included a field experience component in which the students would visit the homes of patients with various afflictions. The student nurses were assigned to families for one day a week for a period of six weeks. I'm sure Dr. Gnade, and the nursing staff at Grady Hospital, recommended Howdy and I be part of the student's learning experience. I still suspected the professional medical community knew little about Alzheimer's, so it seemed to me the disease would be totally new for most of the student nurses.

I felt honored Howdy and I were picked. The whole experience turned out to be a positive one for us, and I believe for the student nurses as well. We were chosen two years in a row, so I felt as if we were twice blessed. The first year a young lady named Nancy Sherman was our helper, and the second year it was a young lady named Heather Nardin. We became very good friends with both young women. I learned a lot from them, and I believe they learned a lot from Howdy and me.

Both young women asked me a lot of questions about my feelings as I cared for Howdy. I always tried to be honest with them, and so I explained my feelings at that time were quite different from what they were in the beginning of Howdy's illness. I agreed to tell them whatever they wanted to know. I felt they needed to know what I was thinking, and what emotions I was feeling in different situations. Howdy couldn't tell them what was going on in his head, so it was all up to me. I told them in the beginning I was very angry about the things Howdy would do and at times I couldn't control my anger, but over time, I did learn to control my emotions. I changed into a calm and understanding person – it took time, but I did manage to change for the better. That was the first experience with an Alzheimer's patient and a full-time caregiver in a home environment, for both of them. They said they truly appreciated my candor.

One of the things I shared with them was the way Howdy's mood could change so dramatically in no time at all. One day for example, Howdy and I were in our bedroom. I had a small round pillow I put under my legs to help me sleep at night and Howdy picked it up off the bed, handed it to me, and said, "Here's your ball." We laughed about it, and he appeared to be in a really jovial mood. That afternoon, we were sitting on the couch. Howdy tried to get up, but he just couldn't make it by himself. I stood up, took both of his hands in mine, and started to pull him up. Suddenly, his feet slipped out from under him, and he fell back into the chair. Either he thought I'd pushed him, or I didn't hold on to him tightly enough to keep him from falling. Very angrily he yelled, "You pushed me!" I tried to tell him he'd slipped, but he didn't want to accept my explanation. He stayed mad at me for a long time after that. Now I look back on it, whenever Howdy fell, or hurt himself, he always wanted to blame me.

One day, I could tell Howdy was in a bad mood because nothing I did for him was done to his satisfaction. So when one of the nurses, Bev Wertz, came to take care of him, I knew she was in for a rough time. She didn't have any trouble getting Howdy into the shower, but he wasn't very happy with her. He grumbled about everything she did, from the temperature of the water, to the amount of soap she was using. Some days it seemed as if he just had to gripe about something, and that was definitely one of those days. When she bathed him, she always saved his head for last. As she was running water over his head to rinse it, he suddenly screamed, "That's enough, damn it! Are you going to drown me, or what?" It was a pleasant surprise to hear Howdy's voice, because he rarely ever talked to anyone other than me, let alone yell at anyone. Bev and I got a lot of enjoyment from him that day. Several times, as the day went on, I looked at him and said "I can't believe you talked so much today." He just looked at me and grinned.

One of the most difficult things for me to do was to make important decisions by myself. For example, I'd given a great deal of thought to getting Howdy a hospital bed. Finally, after he fell out of bed several times one night, my mind was made up. I'd exhausted all the resources I could find to keep him from falling out, but nothing seemed to work. As it turned out, deciding to get the bed was the easy part, the most difficult part was figuring out where to put it. My first thought was to get rid of our bed, and put the hospital bed in our bedroom. After thinking it over, however, I decided to put it in the living room. I knew having the bed in the bedroom would keep me from paying attention to Howdy as much as I should, as he was spending more and more time in bed. So, I opted to have the hospital bed set up where I could interact with him, no matter what I was doing.

With Howdy right there in the middle of the living room, I was with him all the time. He could hear my voice, and see me, and know I was near. Every time I passed him, I made a point of speaking to him. If he'd have been in another room, I wouldn't have spoken to him nearly as often. That arrangement worked out very well. To ensure I'd be near Howdy round the clock, I began sleeping on the living room couch, and I eventually slept there for more than three years. During that time, I became a very light sleeper. The couch opened up to a queen sized bed, but there wasn't very much room in the living room when I opened it all the way. Consequently, I didn't open it up. Over time, I adjusted to sleeping on that narrow couch.

One of the problems Howdy was experiencing at that time was trouble swallowing water, but not solid food. I wondered why that was. I asked the doctors, but they didn't have an answer that satisfied me. I started to think about it quite a bit, and finally, came up with my own reason why. I figured he could grasp the solid foods with his tongue and control them. The liquids just slipped right by, so he couldn't control them. Whatever the reason, Howdy had problems choking on liquids. I never convinced anyone about my little theory, but I was convinced my diagnosis was correct. I lived with the disease day in and day out, and most of the time, I had to reason things out for myself. The doctors only saw Howdy once in a while, but I could observe what he did first hand. Being convinced I knew more about Howdy than anyone else gave me the courage to make most of the difficult decisions on my own.

At least, I didn't have to wrestle with the decision about whether to stay in Florida or Ohio anymore. When March came that year, it was so nice not to have a house to close up in Florida, friends to say good-bye to, and a long and arduous trip to navigate back to Ohio – we were already there!

Another blessing with being in Ohio permanently was Harry no longer came to stay with us for months at a time, but he did visit us quite often. That really worked out better for all of us, as we didn't get on each other's nerves as much during a short stay. About the time we were getting in each other's way, he'd be gone, and the next time we saw him, we were glad to have him stay again. From that point on, when he visited, he usually stayed from four days to a week. Another good thing that happened at that time was Harry finally beginning to realize Howdy was not putting on an act about his illness. Harry had always been so good to me through the years, and I truly didn't want there to be hard feelings between us. So, when he admitted to me Howdy wasn't fooling, it was like someone lifted a huge weight off my shoulders. I can't tell you how very happy that made me.

The coming of spring that year brought even more time for me to work on getting things in shape outside. Every year we lived in the trailer in Delaware, I seemed to find more room to plant additional flowers and bushes around the house. I loved digging in the earth, and to be able to look up at the patio and see Howdy sitting peacefully in a chair, as I puttered around with my landscaping, was delightful. It seemed to me Howdy liked to watch me digging and planting, too. When we lived in Brunswick, Howdy had a rose garden where he liked to plant all the latest Jackson and Perkins roses. He really loved that garden. But, for as much as Howdy loved roses, I didn't want the bother of taking care of rose bushes, so I never planted any. Howdy never told me if he was disappointed or not. Actually, I wasn't even sure he knew we had a garden.

Whenever the Bevers came up from South Carolina to visit their families in Aliquippa, they'd always swing by Delaware to spend two or three days with us. Howdy and I were no longer able to make it down to South Carolina, so it was nice we were still able to see them each year. However, after their visit that particular summer, I didn't know if John would ever allow them to come again. It was a particularly hot summer, and John was especially grateful for the shade from the trees just outside his bedroom window. Usually, one of the benefits of having the Bevers visit was their willingness to help out around the trailer doing little jobs for us. So, one morning, while John was off on one of his frequent road trips for his job, Jim decided the three flowering crab trees I'd planted outside John's bedroom window should be thinned out. Jim got right to work early that morning and started sawing and cutting. By the time John got home that afternoon, almost every bit of shade he'd enjoyed from those trees was gone. His room was hotter than hell, and he was hopping mad. For the rest of that summer, temperatures soared almost every day, and poor John sweltered with no shade from the trees for relief. I know deep down inside, John loved the Bevers just as much as we did, and now whenever we get together, we have a good laugh about that incident, but for a brief time that summer, I thought John was going to kill Jim.

Chuck and Aileen Grof, our next-door neighbors from the trailer park in Dade City, stopped for a couple of days on their way back to Florida from Michigan that summer, too. You'd have thought we hadn't seen each other for years the way we talked and talked. We laughed because they were driving one of the longest R.Vs. I'd ever seen. Parked out front, it looked as if it were as long as our mobile home. I don't know how they manipulated it on the narrow streets of the park, but somehow they did. They stayed overnight, and we talked well into the evening and got caught up on the news concerning all of our friends in Florida. What a delightful visit we had!

Later that summer, we had a visit from some other friends from Florida, but that was not a pleasant experience. They came for a visit, and stayed for a couple of hours. We had a nice lunch and caught up on the news of more of our friends in Florida. I didn't realize it at the time, but somewhere in the conversation, I made a remark that came back to haunt me for some time thereafter. I was at one of those low points in my caring for Howdy, a day when the pain and frustrations of that terrible disease seemed overwhelming, and I couldn't cope with it anymore. Foolishly, I said I was mad at God for all the suffering he allowed Howdy to endure with Alzheimer's. I also explained I knew those feelings wouldn't last, but at the moment, what I said was an honest statement of how I felt. I stressed it was something I had to work out between God and myself. Well, after they returned to Florida, I received an awful letter from the lady telling me how extremely disappointed she was in me. She went on to say she was very sorry she'd ever prayed for me, and she'd never waste any more prayers on me, thereafter.

I was so mad, so upset, and disgusted I planned to write her a nasty letter in reply, asking her if that was the Christian attitude she espoused. How could she so easily turn her back on a friend, under the trying circumstance I was going through, and still call herself a Christian? But after writing a few lines, I decided she wasn't worth getting upset over, and I never finished the letter. I finally decided she needed more help than I did. Eventually, I did get over being mad at God, after God and I worked it out.

August 1991

By the time we reached the late summer of 1991, Howdy was choking on liquids more and more, but solid foods still didn't seem to give him any trouble at all. I wondered if the liquids were getting into his lungs and causing problems. Was that the reason why he had congestive heart failure so much? I think it was, but none of his doctors ever told me that.

Howdy went into the hospital again with congestive heart failure in August of 1991. After much deliberation, I finally agreed with the two surgeons from Grady Hospital who recommended while Howdy was in there, he should have a feeding tube inserted into his stomach. There were a lot of pros and cons about putting a tube into someone's stomach. It took a lot of soul searching for me to come to a decision about that. I'll never know for sure if I made the right decision or not. But I like to think I did, and that decision allowed me to have Howdy for a couple more years. I certainly didn't want him to choke to death. It was times like that when I wished God would come down from Heaven and tell me the right thing to do. It would've been a lot easier. Deep down, even during those darkest of times, I think I continued to hope Howdy would get better, although common sense told me it wasn't going to be.

I don't know what I might've decided if I'd have waited a while before making the decision about the feeding tube. Would I have said "yes," or "no"? So much happened over the next few months, I really don't know what I'd have done. I just might've changed my mind. All Howdy had to do was look at me with his big, soulful eyes, or burst into one of his ear-to-ear grins, and I melted. Love sometimes clouded my judgment, but on the other hand, it made everything easier.

By the day of the operation, I'd convinced myself we were doing the right thing for Howdy. After the operation the doctors came to me, and said they had a bad time of it. Howdy had three quarters of his stomach removed when he had the bleeding ulcer in 1949. Naturally, his stomach was much smaller than it should have been. I guess I assumed his stomach would grow larger again, so I never said anything to the doctors before they inserted the tube. Also, I thought they'd see the scars and realize he'd gone through a major operation on his stomach. By not telling them, however, I almost caused a serious problem for the doctors. Fortunately, the operation went well, and Howdy made a complete recovery. As long as everything came out all right, no harm was done. That hospital stay lasted ten days.

For more than a year, we only had to use the tube for liquids. During that time, Howdy handled the solid foods very well. Eventually, I did have to put his food through a blender. As long as I pureed the food, he handled it okay. He still loved the taste of food, and I loved making it for him. I got a big kick out of figuring out what different combinations of foods would taste good being pureed together.

Thereafter, when Howdy had bad days, I blamed myself. But on those wonderful days, when he touched me so very tenderly, I knew I'd been doing the right thing all along. I always hoped and prayed God understood my selfishness for wanting to keep Howdy with me for as long as I could.

CHAPTER 23 – JANEAN

Fall of 1991

Our granddaughter, Janean, began attending Wittenberg University in Springfield, Ohio, in the fall of 1991. During one of her freshman classes, the subject of putting an elderly person in a home came up. Most of the students said they'd never do that. But my granddaughter said, "Listen to me, and I'll tell you about my grandmother. After you hear this story, you might think differently about what you'd do in the same situation."

She proceeded to tell them about some of the things I'd gone through. Mostly she stressed I was a prisoner in my own house. I guess that was the best way for her to describe my situation, because she was struck by the fact there was no way I could go out and leave Howdy alone whenever I wanted to. If I absolutely had to go out for groceries, or other essential items, I always had to have someone come in to take care of him, even for a short run to the store.

Janean told her classmates I never had the luxury of deciding on the spur of the moment if I wanted to go shopping. And the one or two hours a day I had someone come in from Monday through Thursday weren't very much. But, on Friday, I had four hours all to myself. I felt like I was on vacation. I made the most of the time I had by rushing from one store to another to get everything done. Some days, I got my shopping finished, other days I didn't. There never seemed to be enough time to do everything.

Janean also stressed to her classmates at any time of the day or night I could be putting a load of wash in the washer, or getting out the bucket and a lot of rags to start scrubbing the floors to cleanup a mess.

She said it was good I didn't seem to mind doing it, even though there were many times when I couldn't finish a meal, or even take a quick nap when I'd been up half the night because Howdy needed attention.

Janean told them there were many times when I thought Howdy was dying. The spells of choking were the scariest. At least when he was choking, I could help him to get relief. But, for most of the other problems he encountered, I had to figure out what the problem was first.

Putting someone in a nursing home, she added, is not always an option, but under certain circumstances, it's a necessity. If circumstances warranted putting someone in a home, and there wasn't any other way out - it might have to be done.

She went on to explain you just can't leave someone with Alzheimer's alone to go to work, or to go out for the evening with friends. The chances of them setting the house on fire, or some other disaster happening is too great. People who are suffering from the disease are so childlike - they have no sense of right or wrong.

Janean told the class to think about all of those things, and if they ever had to make that type of decision, they'd have a better understanding of how their decision will impact family members who may become full-time caregivers. She said one of the things in my favor was the age difference between Howdy and me. The eleven-and-a-half years didn't seem like a lot, but I'd never have been able to handle him if we'd been closer in age. Also, I was retired, and had no job to take up a lot of my time.

At the end of her speech, Janean stressed every person's circumstances are different, and each person has to do what their circumstances allow them to do.

December 1991

By the end of 1991, Howdy was talking less and less, and I was having more one-way conversations. Sometimes, I couldn't believe I was doing all that talking. I really thought Howdy could hear what I was saying to him, but I couldn't be sure he understood a single word. Most of the time, he seemed like he was listening, because he'd have different expressions on his face depending on what I said. I could even get a hearty laugh out of him from time to time when I said something funny.

Occasionally, I'd ask him to hold my hands when I talked to him, thinking somehow that would make him understand me. There were times when he'd wiggle his fingers, or move his hands, or squeeze my hand, which convinced me I was on the right track. I always made a point of looking people in the eye when I talked to them, so it wasn't unusual for me to keep looking into Howdy's big, brown eyes during my conversations with him.

Somehow, with all the congestion in our living room we managed to squeeze in a Christmas tree that holiday season, which delighted Howdy. Whenever the tree lights were on, his face would light up, and he could hardly take his eyes off that tree. I felt as if Howdy could sense the excitement in the air, and in his way, he enjoyed the holidays as much as we did. That year, I didn't leave the tree up as long as I had in the past. But when it was gone, I think Howdy really missed the lights.

Also that year, we were very fortunate to make it through the holidays without any major incidents. Shortly after Christmas, however, Howdy started acting strangely, and I knew he was getting sick again. He started coughing quite a bit, but he wasn't running a temperature. Then all of a sudden, on a Saturday, Howdy had a temperature of 99.6. I called the nurse, and she came right over. She didn't hear any grating in his lungs, just a loud rattle in his chest. By then Howdy was coughing up a lot of phlegm, and moaning as if he were in a lot of pain. We decided to call an ambulance to take him to the hospital.

It turned out Howdy was quite ill with congestive heart failure. He was hospitalized for five days, and with some of the other problems he was having, we were afraid he might not make it. That time, like so many other times when we thought he wouldn't respond to the treatment he was receiving, he fooled all of us. Miraculously, he suddenly began looking healthy again.

Another problem surfaced on that visit to the hospital - bedsores. He went into the hospital without any bedsores, but when he came out, he had three. There were two sores on his buttocks, and another one at the end of his spine. That was the first time I'd ever seen a bedsore, and I had no idea how to care for them. I had to learn very quickly how to deal with them, however. Somehow, I was under the impression in a few weeks we'd cure the sores and that would be the end of them - another daydream of mine went away in a hurry. No matter what we tried, we were never able to get rid of them completely.

I kept wondering why he suddenly had bedsores. Then I remembered his mother telling me when he was about five years old he had a very bad case of the deadly influenza that was sweeping the country at that time. He almost died. He was in the hospital when his mother discovered three of the worse bedsores imaginable. She immediately wrapped him in a blanket, and took him home without the doctor's permission. The hospital tried to persuade her to bring him back, and warned her if she didn't, he'd die. But she lovingly nursed him at home and he recovered. Consequently, Howdy had the deep scars of that illness all of his life - one on each hip, and one at the base of his spine. The doctor explained to me the dead tissue of a bedsore tends to develop very quickly. That was the major reason why we were never able to get rid of them completely.

While Howdy was in the hospital, Mary Jane and Jess came up from Pennsylvania again and stayed for several weeks. They were always a big help with Howdy. I just don't know what I would've done without them during those difficult times. I do believe there's an angel in all of us, and especially in the souls of those people who are born caregivers. Mary Jane and I spent so much time at the hospital we were grateful when Jess always had lunch or supper ready for us – another one of our angels.

That trip to the hospital made me realize I needed to work harder at taking care of Howdy, but I didn't mind. They inserted a catheter in him in the hospital, which served as a warning system because I was able to see the color of his urine. I could also watch for sediment in his urine. Those types of visual checks were much better than taking frequent blood tests. For as long as he had a catheter in him, we didn't have very many problems with it.

A few weeks later, Howdy began acting strangely again. Every time I got close to him, he'd grab me and pull me toward him. His mouth was moving a mile a minute. He was desperately trying to tell me something, but only garbled sounds were coming out. I felt terrible because I couldn't understand him. It was amazing how strong he was, given each day he was in bed, he lost a little more weight. But when he pulled me toward him, I could hardly pull away. Eventually, he relaxed his grip, and when he let go, I wondered what was so important. That scenario repeated itself every so often, and I always felt so terribly helpless.

February 15, 1992

Just when I thought I'd never hear Howdy's voice again, he suddenly began talking up a storm one day. How could he go from not talking at all, to being so talkative? That was another thing I could never figure out.

It was the middle of February, normally a very depressing time in Ohio because of all the dreary weather, but Howdy was in a really good mood. After bathing him one particular morning, I went into the kitchen to make him breakfast. He was in the living room, and I could see him across the kitchen counter. He was lying in the hospital bed watching me. All of a sudden, he yelled "Hey, you! What do you think you're doing?" We laughed as I carried his tray of food into him. I explained he wouldn't get any food if I didn't take the time to fix it. He seemed to accept that explanation and then he ate the entire meal. His appetite was always good, so I hardly ever had to coax him to eat.

Howdy had false teeth and he always had trouble with his lower plate, because he didn't like to use any type of denture adhesive and the plate slipped around in his mouth. With that in mind, I began to wonder if he might have a problem with the plate slipping in such a way he'd choke on the plate when I wasn't around to prevent him from choking to death. So, I made the decision to take his dentures out of his mouth and I never put them back in again. But I didn't want him to have trouble chewing his food, so I decided to grind up everything I fed him. It became quite a challenge for me to come up with different combinations of ground up foods that were also tasty for him.

Thereafter, he began to eat much bigger breakfasts than he usually did. I was pleased, as I wanted to make sure he got plenty of nourishing foods. I had the feeling Howdy's good appetite helped him to live longer than he might have if he had refused to eat. He enjoyed food, especially for someone who'd become quite thin and I enjoyed the challenge of coming up with different menus. The food not only had to smell good, but it also had to look good and be tasteful. I tried putting several foods together. Being able to make such a variety of different ground-up meals really helped a lot. I'd never have guessed a small food chopper would be the most used mechanical device in the kitchen – but it was.

I found myself thinking of food more and more. Some of the combinations I came up with were pretty inventive, I thought. For example, I'd make a piece of toast, then poach an egg, add several spoons of peanut butter, and occasionally add some fruit. Then I'd grind them all up. Or I'd cook some oatmeal with fruit (bananas or peaches), and some peanut butter. I think peanut butter gave it a sweet taste. Coming up with different ideas was pretty easy. Lunches and suppers were easier than breakfast. Howdy would eat whatever I made for supper, as long as I ground everything up for him. Cake and Jell-O were different, however. There was no need for grinding because Howdy had no trouble swallowing those items. They just melted in his mouth. Applesauce was another one of his favorite treats.

I didn't have any trouble pulling Howdy up in his bed when the two of us were alone. I always liked to keep Howdy's head elevated, so he could breathe easier and see what was going on around him better. Therefore, I raised the head of his bed, which put the bed on a slant. That caused gravity to gradually make him slide down and end up with his feet against the bottom of the bed. When that happened, I had to go to the head of the bed, get a good grip on the draw sheet, and slowly pull it up. A draw sheet is an extra narrow blanket you can pull to move the patient around on. Usually, Howdy would just move up with the sheet. After doing that several times, we'd run out of extra draw sheet. At those times, it'd be a big project getting him up in the bed, so I'd climb up, straddle him, and place my hands under both of his arms. I always told him to help me as much as he could. Then I'd lift and pull him toward the head of the bed, stopping when I thought he was high enough. Sometimes, we could get through the ordeal rather quickly. Other times, it'd take several attempts to get him where he needed to be. As long as I didn't have an asthma attack in the middle of the procedure, all was well. I always tried to explain to him what I was planning to do because I didn't want to scare him. Then I'd yell, "alley-oop" and start to lift him up using all my strength. I always encouraged him to help by pushing with his feet. He really couldn't do that, but we got a good laugh out of it anyhow.

Since the bed was right next to a window, I often thought of what would happen if I fell out of the window during one of those sessions. I asked Howdy what he'd do. He thought that was very funny, and he started to laugh. I started to laugh, too, and we had a good time sharing a hearty chuckle.

I often thought of how funny it'd be to someone else. We must have been quite a sight, me standing on the bed, which was very unsteady, and Howdy lying there helplessly. I wouldn't have thought it was very funny had I fallen on top of him. It was very important for me to look on the humorous side of these things, or else I would've been crying too much.

Sometimes, the smallest things would set me to wondering. For example, I'd think about Howdy not being able to scratch his nose, or his head, or any other part of his body. I'd think of the many times I scratched something without giving it a second thought. But there was poor Howdy unable to do even the simplest things like scratching an itch for himself. Once in a while, I'd start scratching his nose then go up to his head. He'd lift up his head as if to say, "Don't forget the back of my head!" Then I'd roll him over and start on his back. The look of contentment that came over his face was great. Just to see him smiling made an incredible feeling of joy come over me. You'd think I was the one getting scratched.

I could always tell whatever I did for Howdy, he appreciated. He'd reach out for me, and try so hard to speak to me. Even when nothing came out, I knew he was trying to thank me.

CHAPTER 24 – HOME CARE

I really can't explain how depressed I became whenever Howdy tried so very hard to tell me something and nothing but gibberish came out. Occasionally, I wondered if I could've changed things in some way if I'd been able to think more clearly myself. Because the world has come so far with electronics I wonder if I'd taped some of Howdy's mutterings if someone might've been able to decipher what he was trying to say to me? Sometimes, we went for days with hardly a peep out of Howdy, and then all of a sudden, he'd try to talk. As the year went on, we noticed Howdy was talking less and less.

Throughout 1992 we struggled along. Howdy had some good days here and there, but unfortunately, he also had some very bad days. We had another scare on June 25th of that year. Howdy started having difficulty breathing, so I called the medics. As soon as they arrived and heard the rattling and congestion in his chest, they rushed him to the hospital. I immediately called Mary Jane in Pennsylvania and drove to the hospital to be with Howdy. The doctors in the emergency room decided his condition wasn't bad enough for him to be admitted, so after four hours of treatment they sent us home. Once again, we had to give Howdy more antibiotics. I was so busy taking care of Howdy I neglected to call Mary Jane back to tell her to cancel her trip. But as it turned out, this was one of those times when Howdy and I really needed her and Jess.

By the time Mary Jane and Jess arrived, Howdy was almost too much for me to handle. They pitched right in and we got to work taking care of him. The doctors in the emergency room at the hospital had gotten Howdy's breathing under control, so we turned our attention to his other increasingly serious problem - bedsores. No matter what we did for them they just seemed to get worse. We went into a routine of changing the bandages on the bedsores three or four times a day, and we also tried turning him quite often. None of that seemed to make much of a difference. He moaned and groaned in such a pathetic way I just wanted to start crying again.

When he coughed, he'd really yell, too. He must've been in a lot of pain. I couldn't believe how much phlegm he coughed up at one time. I had some sticks with sponges on the ends that were absolutely wonderful. They were about six or eight inches long - much longer than a normal swab. Because of their extra length, I could reach to the back of his throat, twisting and pulling in a circle until the sponges caught hold of the phlegm. Then, I'd keep pulling till it was all out. Throughout the entire procedure, I was extremely apprehensive, fearing I'd panic and not be able to do what I had to do calmly. I always had the fear Howdy would choke to death while we were in the midst of this ordeal, and it'd be my fault because I didn't clear his airway quickly enough. That was another good reason why I couldn't leave Howdy alone.

After each of those sessions, Howdy seemed to be worn out, and he'd have a terrible look on his face. I tried to explain everything to him, but I was never sure he understood what I was trying to tell him.

On one of the nurse's regular days to visit, she examined Howdy, and after listening to his chest, she called the doctor. After talking to the nurse, the doctor ordered a portable chest X-ray unit to come to the house.

Luckily, there was no pneumonia at that time. But the nurse decided something wasn't right with Howdy's urine, and she wondered if he might have a bladder infection. So, she took a urine sample and had it tested. It took three days for the culture to be analyzed, and when it was, it came out positive - he definitely had an infection. The tests showed Howdy had something growing in his urine - as if he didn't have enough troubles already! The next step was to find the correct antibiotic to kill it. Early the next morning I found another small bedsore starting on his back. I immediately started working on it, and thankfully, I was eventually able to get it under control.

On the following Saturday, Howdy's urine was clearer than it had been for a long time. The medicine was doing the trick! Just when we had one worry taken care of, however, we changed the bandages on Howdy's bedsores, and I thought they looked awful. But the nurse thought they looked a little better. I figured she knew a lot more about it than I did, because she saw patients with bedsores all the time. She measured them and said they were a little smaller than the last time she measured them.

I became so conscious of bedsores, and how hard they were to treat, the moment I saw the smallest lesion on his skin I had it checked out. Fortunately, all of our helpful nurses knew what the danger signals were, too, and we were all on the alert to anything different that appeared on Howdy's skin. So, when something looked the least bit odd to any of us, we'd all check it out. I was impressed with how fast some of the medicines could cure something, and how well the doctors and nurses were trained to know just what to do.

I had a habit of taking Howdy's temperature quite often, and it amazed me how it could fluctuate so rapidly. One hour it would be 98.2 degrees, and the next hour it could jump up to 101.4, or higher. For that reason, I felt justified in taking his temperature frequently.

After staying for almost two and a half weeks, my two angels, Mary Jane and Jess, went home again. Somehow, Howdy must've known they were gone, because he was very uneasy. That entire day he was very flushed, but his urine was clear. It seemed to be a good day for coughing. He started to cough early in the day, and I didn't think he'd ever stop. He coughed on and off all day long. At bedtime, I gave him a cold pill and more cough medicine. We finally got to sleep around midnight.

The next morning, I guess the medicine hadn't quite worn off, because Howdy didn't want to eat his breakfast. That was unusual, but he just kept falling back asleep. Around lunchtime, he finally woke up - ravenously hungry.

Some mornings, Howdy would wake up and not be hungry at all. After several hours of not eating, his appetite would return, and I could tell he was himself again. He'd almost gulp his food down.

Howdy had diarrhea quite often, so we became well acquainted with Lomotil. It worked pretty well most of the time, but there were times when nothing seemed to work – even Lomotil.

Howdy always seemed to either sleep too much, or not enough. When he slept a lot, I blamed the medicines – even though I was very grateful to have them. After all, wasn't medicine supposed to relax someone? I always figured if you were relaxed enough you'd fall asleep pretty easily.

It was amazing how Howdy could go from sleeping most of the time to hardly sleeping at all, especially when he was being given the same medications all the time. It seemed as if Howdy would go through a spell where he slept most of the day for days at a time. That always seemed to be followed by several days when he'd stay awake for extended periods. I just had to be flexible enough to adjust to his sleep/wake pattern, so I could cope with the situation. I always tried to sleep when he did, and stay awake when he was awake. When I showed patience and restraint, I asked myself, "Is that really me?" For most of my life, I was as impatient as a person could possibly be, but then, when I had to be patient – I was.

One morning, when I woke up, I noticed there wasn't any urine in Howdy's bag. As I often did under such circumstances, I started to panic before I got my wits about myself and figured out what was going on. I decided to keep a good eye on the bag, and give it until about ten o'clock, to see what happened. Slowly, but surely the bag started to fill up. If he hadn't urinated by ten, I'd have given him a Lasix pill. That situation was a good example of how far I'd come as a caregiver. I'd progressed to the point where I tried to solve any problems that came up on my own before I called a nurse or the doctor. And there were many instances when, one way or another, I'd figure it out on my own. I'm sure the medical professionals appreciated me not calling them ten times a day over trivial matters, although there were days when I was tempted to do that.

Every once in a while, Howdy would vomit, and I was sure it was because of all the medicine he was taking. So, I tried to figure out how to give him the medicine in a way that wouldn't upset his stomach. I decided I should give him his medicine in smaller amounts, and that seemed to help. When he belched a lot, I'd give him a small amount of anti-acid, and that seemed to work, too.

I always made sure to read the directions on Howdy's medicines. Most of them stated they should be given with food or milk. So, I made sure I always did what the directions called for, but that didn't always work. Occasionally, he'd have an upset stomach after I gave him a certain medication. I could tell by the expression on his face something was wrong with him. If he felt all right, he'd smile a lot, and if not, he certainly knew how to frown.

We began treating Howdy's bedsores with a wash of half-saltwater and half-peroxide a couple times a day. Then we decided to keep his bandages wet with a saltwater solution. We always carefully covered the sores with bandages after we cleaned the wounds. Finally, after several weeks of following that routine, I thought the sores were looking better than they'd looked for a long time.

With the beginning of another school year at Ohio Wesleyan it was time for nurses to begin training once again. Much to my surprise, Howdy and I were again picked for a student nurse to come once a week for six weeks. The student nurse was to learn from us, and we were to learn from her. Once again, that was a wonderful experience for us. The fact we'd been chosen for the second time made me feel quite important.

I was beginning to feel like a teacher. It was such a good feeling to explain to our new student about all of the ups and downs of taking care of an Alzheimer's patient. I not only told her about the bad times, but I also made sure to tell her about the good times as well. I tried to let her become privy to my thought processes, so she had a better understanding of where I was coming from. I believe she got as much out of those visits as I did. I always felt I had a lot to share with others.

Once again, Howdy contracted bronchitis and had to be admitted to the hospital for eleven days, from September 4th until September 14th. As usual, Mary Jane and Jess came to help. It seemed like we made quite a few trips to the hospital that year because Howdy was in the hospital more in 1992, than any other year.

It was good Howdy's illness wasn't pneumonia this time, but having bronchitis wasn't a good thing either. And just when it looked like Howdy was starting to improve, he came up with some new problems. As if common bronchitis wasn't bad enough by itself, the doctors found three different types of bacteria growing in his lungs, kidneys, and bladder. After hearing that news, I was close to despair, because it sounded as if his situation was hopeless this time. Then suddenly, he showed improvement. He improved so much, in fact, the doctor told us Howdy could go home the next day. Why I always got excited when I received the news Howdy was going home, I'll never know, but I think Mary Jane, Jess, and I were exhausted from spending so much time at the hospital. That's why it was such a great disappointment when, after the doctor said he could go home, the next morning Howdy spiked a fever, and that meant he had to stay a few days longer.

After that particularly difficult relapse, Doctor Gnade decided it was time for us to have a conference about Howdy. So, the next day, we had our chat. The doctor told me Howdy wasn't responding to the treatment, and he, again, wanted me to consider very seriously putting him in a nursing home. I think he could tell what a toll Howdy's condition was taking on me, but I simply couldn't put him in a home. And I think I finally convinced Doctor Gnade I could never do that. I explained to him Mary Jane and I would be at the nursing home early each morning anyhow to bathe Howdy, shave him, clean his teeth and mouth, brush his hair, and whatever else needed to be done. We might as well do it in our own home where we had all of the supplies we needed. Even though he disagreed with my decision, he knew I was determined to have it my way, and he finally said, "All right."

Because Howdy's blood count was very low at that time, Dr. Gnade decided he'd need a blood transfusion before he could go home. But after a few more tests, his blood count went back up, so he changed his mind and decided a transfusion wasn't needed. A couple days later, however, when Howdy was to come home, his blood count went down again. This time Dr. Gnade ordered the transfusion after all. After the transfusion, Howdy was more alert than usual - he was like a new person. It wasn't as if I thought I knew more than the doctors, but I tried to convince them Howdy's reaction to that transfusion made a great change in his attitude and his ability to perform certain motor skills. Because I was with him all the time, I was able to observe his reaction to whatever they gave him. The doctors and nurses saw him only briefly, but I was with him constantly, that's why I was convinced the transfusion had the same effect as a wonder drug of some sort.

While Howdy was in the hospital that time, he seemed to reach a point where there was really nothing more any of us could do for him. We just tried to make things a little easier for him, such as ordering a better mattress for his bed. Finally, Dr. Gnade announced he'd decided to send Howdy home the following Monday. I had to sign some papers releasing the hospital and doctors of any responsibility, but with a promise I'd get all the help I needed. Thereafter, the wonderful nurses were our "doctors" because the doctor didn't make house calls. I knew the only time I'd see the doctor would be if Howdy went back into the hospital, or if I went to see him for an appointment for myself, or talked to him on the phone. On those occasions when I did call Dr. Gnade, he never cut me short, and he always had time for me to "cry on his shoulder."

From that point on, every time something went wrong, I couldn't figure out on my own, I called the doctor. He was always very helpful, especially considering he wasn't getting paid for any of the time he spent on the phone talking to me. I never had the feeling he didn't want to be bothered with my problems. I must say of all the doctors we dealt with during Howdy's illness my favorite was Doctor Gnade. I also came to regard him, and the many nurses, as my friends.

I just can't stress enough how much we came to depend on and appreciate the nurses who cared for Howdy. Most amazing to me were the student nurses who did everything the regular nurses did. On Thursdays, they'd come and take Howdys' vital signs, temperature, blood pressure, etc. Then they'd give Howdy a bath, change his bandages, and put clean linens on his bed. They did just about everything that had to be done to make him comfortable. It wasn't easy giving someone a bath when that person couldn't help in any way. Every movement was up to the bather. I jokingly referred to him as my eighty-year-old baby. By then, he was pathetically thin and weighed less than a hundred pounds. Even so, for someone trying to move him around, it was a strenuous task, because he was dead weight. It usually took me anywhere from an hour, to an hour and a half, just to give him his bath. It sometimes took the nurses longer than that.

Taking care of Howdy's bedsores continued to be one of the hardest things for me to do. I increased the amount of time I spent on treating the bedsores, and some days I worked on them four times, or more. Bandages and salves were a must in our house. The bedsores had pockets under the skin that had to be washed out with long Q-tips, rinsed, and salved before applying new bandages. As long as we explained to Howdy what we were doing, and did things slowly enough so he could understand, he seemed to relax and let us do what we had to do.

CHAPTER 25 – CLINITRON BED

We gradually transformed our living room into a hospital room filled with nursing supplies including Howdy's medications, salves, bandages, and bed linens as the year 1992 went along. It was essential everything we needed be within arm's reach for when we needed something in a hurry. Unfortunately, the emergencies were becoming more frequent, and there wasn't always enough time to go into another room for the needed items.

It seemed as if we were washing Howdy off and changing the bed linens more and more often. I'm not sure Sears and Roebuck expected their washers and dryers to be used to such an extent in a private home. At just about any hour of the day or night, we were putting bed linens, etc., into the washer and dryer.

Howdy must have had the cleanest body of anyone in the city of Delaware. His skin should have been silky smooth with all of the lotions we used on him. Later, when his skin started to peel off, the nurses and doctors explained a lot of it had to do with nutrition. Even though I thought I was feeding him really good meals, and his appetite was still good, it evidently wasn't enough.

The fall of 1992 wasn't too eventful, but that didn't mean it wasn't stressful. We were always on the alert for any emergency that might arise. One morning, after a fairly good night's sleep, I woke up as usual and went over to Howdy's bed to check on him and received a terrible shock. As I stepped onto the floor next to Howdy's bed, my bare feet landed in an icy cold pool of liquid that gushed between my toes. I looked down at my feet to discover I was standing in a puddle of urine. The catheter bag had somehow broken in the middle of the night, and had leaked all over the floor. Talk about panic! In a matter of seconds, I was kneeling on the floor trying to absorb the urine with a handful of bath towels. I partially filled a small bucket several times as I wrung out the towels. Then, after getting the rug partially dry, I started scrubbing and disinfecting everything to get rid of the smell and the urine. I can't remember how many towels I used, but once again, the washer and dryer went on overtime. Poor Howdy probably wondered what I was doing down on the floor so long. As soon as I finished cleaning up the mess, I got in touch with the nurse and told her to bring a new catheter with her on her next visit. During the entire time Howdy used a catheter, that was the only time a bag broke. When our long ordeal finally ended, one of the first things I did was replace that rug and the padding. Why the house never smelled was a mystery to me, but I guess if you clean thoroughly enough, you can get rid of almost any odor.

By late September of 1992, I still didn't think we were making enough progress with Howdy's bed sores. At that time, I found out about a bed on the market called a Clinitron. According to the brochure I received from one of the nurses, "It is an air fluidized therapy unit designed to treat advanced pressure sores, flaps, grafts, and burns. The system employs the principles of small-particle fluidization to achieve all the properties of a fluid in a completely dry medium. The resulting artificial fluid provides the benefits of true flotation. It virtually eliminates shear and friction. The Clinitron filter sheet is permeable, allowing the downward flow of fluids away from the patient and the upward flow of 1,250 pounds of warm, gentle air to the patient's skin. This dual action prevents the softening of tissue often caused by prolonged exposure to moisture. Thus keeping healthy skin warm and dry." In other words, it used a very fine sand-like substance to simulate a type of waterbed that eliminated a great deal of the pressure around bedsores. I figured it was certainly worth a try - especially when I found out our insurance would help pay for it. So, I decided to order the bed and we waited eagerly to have it delivered.

When the bed arrived, it looked like a big bathtub on a stand. It had to be filled with a ton of non-toxic silicone-coated beads (microspheres). The deliverymen brought the bed into the house empty. Then they carried the beads in by buckets. When I realized how heavy the bed would be, I was quite worried about the possibility that the bed could break through the floor of our house trailer. Since the weight was evenly distributed over the full length of the bed, the deliverymen assured me there wasn't any danger of that happening. To my surprise, it never did go through the floor. But whenever I walked over a certain area of the living room after the bed was removed, I thought I felt a depression in the floor.

It was really clever how the bed operated. Air was drawn into the base where it was filtered, heated, and/or cooled as required. Then it was channeled into the tank through a porous diffuser board. The air flowed gently upward through the beads, and that put the beads in motion. The mixture of air and microspheres behaved like a liquid. Eventually, after using the Clintron bed for a while, Howdy's bed sores showed signs of healing. By that time, however, Howdy's health began to fail more rapidly. I only wish I'd found out about the bed sooner. I knew it wouldn't have made a difference in the progress of the Alzheimer's, but Howdy might've been more comfortable.

When we got into November, I went through another period of "feeling sorry for Ruthie" days, because everything seemed to be going wrong. On one particular afternoon, I slipped and fell down all five steps leading to our front porch. Fortunately, I didn't really get hurt, but my ego was damaged. I don't know if it was from the trauma of the fall, or just an emotional time I was going through, but on and off that entire day, I broke into uncontrollable crying jags I just couldn't stop. There didn't seem to be a reason for it, but I seemed to be breaking down like that quite often at that time. I think it must have done some good, because after I had a day like that, I always felt much better. I'd then have a good talk (one sided) with Howdy. Just talking to him was always a wonderful feeling. There were times when I thought he knew exactly what I was saying to him. Then I'd think, "Did he understand me at all?"

As we got closer to the holidays, I wondered whether Howdy would live through them or not. That had been a worry for the past couple of holiday seasons, but this year, Howdy seemed to be slipping further away each day, and the thought I might lose him at anytime, was always in my mind. But we had a fairly good holiday season that year. We got together with family and some friends, and other than the worry about Howdy's deteriorating condition, I thought it went quite well. It was kind of crowded in the living room with the Clintron bed and all of Howdy's supplies taking up most of the room. We put up a smaller Christmas tree, but it was just as effective as a large one. Howdy seemed to enjoy the bright lights and the glistening Christmas balls on the tree. I really thought I could see him smiling a lot more than usual. He was so thin and frail, but I thought his dark brown eyes stood out all the more. Oh, how I loved him!

After Christmas, it was time to take the tree down, put the lights, Christmas balls, and the rest of the trimmings away for another year. I thought Howdy really missed all of the glitter. As he looked around the room, his mouth would be moving as if he wanted to say something. I was sure he was asking about the tree.

Even after Christmas, our house was never in complete darkness because we had nightlights on in several rooms. With the nightlights, I never had to stop to turn on the lights when Howdy coughed and start choking in the middle of the night. I could get to him immediately, and since all of his supplies were within easy reach, I didn't waste much time turning on lights.

When 1992 ended, we celebrated the coming of the New Year, and moved into 1993 with the apprehension of what the year might bring. I was so very glad Howdy had lived to be with us for that Christmas, but I couldn't be sure he'd make it to the next one. I guess it was selfish of me to want him to stay with us longer, but I couldn't help myself. I really loved him, and I loved taking care of him.

Once in a while, Howdy would get the hiccups. There were times when I didn't think he was going to stop. I tried all kinds of remedies to stop him once the hiccups began. Everyone I talked to had a "never-fail" recipe. We tried most of them. What seemed to work best for me was a small teaspoon of sugar. If the sugar didn't work, I'd give him a small amount of Maalox. One, or both, of those remedies worked most of the time.

In February, we experienced another catheter problem. This time it wasn't the bag, however, it was the catheter itself that began leaking where the bag was inserted into his penis. I figured half of Howdy's urine was leaking out, so I called his primary nurse, Ann Sanderson. I came to think of Ann more as a sister than a nurse. A short while later, she arrived, and I told her Howdy had been moaning quite a bit for a couple of days. I was anxious to see if she could figure out what was causing the problem.

The first thing she did was to put in a new catheter. Unfortunately, the new one leaked just as badly as the old one. Ann and I talked for a while and finally decided Howdy was having bladder spasms. Ann called Dr. Gnade and requested medicine to stop the spasms. Before we had a chance to give Howdy the medicine about two or three ounces of something that looked like sand appeared in the tube. We had a hard time getting it to pass through the tube. It finally did pass through, and thereafter, it didn't leak again. We decided not to give Howdy the medicine unless the catheter started leaking again, or he began to moan again. Ann told me, if he were having spasms, he'd be in a lot of pain. That would be my signal to start giving him the medicine.

Once we got through the catheter problem, I noticed Howdy's skin was really getting bad. Even with all the cream we were using on him, his skin felt like leather. At that point, his skin began peeling off in big pieces. Some days he appeared to lose a layer or more of skin each day.

I asked Dr. Gnade about it again, and he repeated what he told me when the problem first appeared - Howdy was not getting the proper nutrition. A big part of the problem concerned Howdy having difficulty swallowing solid food. Thereafter, we started him on Osmolite. Osmolite was a dietary drink, which had a lot of the nutrients Howdy needed. The easiest way to get the

Osmolite into his system was through his feeding tube. Since he already had the tube in his stomach, I was spared having to make the decision to have one put in at that late date. I don't know what I would've done if I had to make that decision at that stage of his disease.

Somehow, I let Howdy's toenails get too long. I knew cutting them would be a problem for me, so I decided to have a podiatrist come to the house and do them. As the podiatrist was filing his nails, Howdy cried out in pain. The podiatrist told me she wasn't hurting him - he was just yelling. I told her he wasn't yelling from the machine cutting him, but because the machine was hot and he thought she was burning him. I don't know why she didn't figure that out on her own, but I'm sure Howdy felt he was being burned. Finally, she allowed the machine to cool off, and when she continued, Howdy didn't yell any more.

Poor, poor, Howdy! I never really knew if I was doing the right thing for him. When I leaned over him and looked into his eyes, I sometimes had the feeling he might've wanted it all to end. But, because he couldn't tell me what he was thinking, I could never be sure. I guess one never gives up hope. On more than one occasion, I wished God really talked to people. I wanted Him to tell me what to do. On my "down" days, I'd look up to the sky and ask God why He was doing this to us. At times, I got so mad I actually sweared at God. Asking Him to do something for Howdy seemed so fruitless. I was so mad. Not because Howdy was dying, but because of the slow, agonizing way in which he was wasting away. For quite some time, I had a big problem with God, and I thought only I could work it out. In time, I did, and of course, when I did, it was with God's help.

Whenever I'd go through one of those periods, I remembered our friend, who portrayed herself as such a devout and pious lady, and how she became so very upset with me when I told her I was mad at God. I thought about her telling me how sorry she was she ever wasted her time praying for me. I also remembered her saying she'd never pray for me again, no matter how bad things got with Howdy. Those were certainly times in my life when I really needed prayers and spiritual help more than any other time. That lady's attitude toward me was particularly stressful. I guess deep down inside I always felt God understood what I was going through, and in time, he'd forgive me. But I'm not sure some people ever did.

I couldn't understand why certain people felt I'd committed an unpardonable sin because I'd gotten mad at God. I know I'm not the only person who's ever been so terribly frustrated by the seemingly cruel way in which a loved one has suffered to feel anger toward God. I've listened to others explain why they were upset with God, and all of them, in time, got over it. Anyway, I know God watches over all of us, and I was sure he understood how a mere mortal, being under so much stress, could cry out to someone, so why not to an understanding and loving God?

I told another friend about my feelings, on one of her visits to our house. Because she was always bragging about what a good Christian she was, I thought she'd understand my torment. But that was a big mistake on my part, because she didn't write to me for several years. Then, when she finally did write at Christmas one year, and told me how her feelings toward me had changed, I decided not to answer her. Today, I'm sorry I wasn't more forgiving, and I never wrote back.

CHAPTER 26 – JOY AND SADNESS

As we went through the summer of 1993, Howdy became increasingly frail and quite often he seemed to be struggling to breathe. He gradually curled up into a fetal position, which made it more and more difficult for us to straighten his legs when we needed to clean him. It really amazed me, with all of his aches and pain, I was still able to get some hearty laughs out of him from time to time. Even with the difficulty of bathing Howdy, and moving him around in his bed, especially when I was alone with him, I could still get him to chuckle despite the terrible pain he was experiencing. But that pitiful body was a different story. As much as we tried to keep him supple, he seemed to get a little stiffer each day. It seemed as if his muscles were progressively getting tighter. The more we tried to move his arms and legs, the more he'd moan. Despite having the wonderful Clinitron bed, it was becoming harder and harder to manipulate Howdy. But it was much easier moving Howdy in the Clinitron bed than it would've been in a regular bed. Before we touched Howdy, we'd always tell him what we were going to do so we didn't stress him any more than necessary. Any sudden movements always made him twitch in alarm. The draw sheets were every bit as handy with the new bed. With a few tugs and flips of the sheets, we were able to roll him over easily to the opposite side from the one we were working on. We always made jokes about how heavy he was to move around, even though he only weighed a mere 100 pounds by that time. I never thought he'd get much thinner, but he did.

It seemed to me Howdy was losing weight at a much faster rate than he had previously, especially when we started him on the Osmolite, and took him off solid foods. Dr. Gnade and the nurses explained he still wasn't getting enough nutrition. The condition of his skin worried me too, but that was also because he wasn't getting enough nutrients. At the same time, I noticed Howdy wasn't moaning and groaning as much as he had before. Whether that was because he was sleeping more or not I didn't know, but I wanted to think he wasn't enduring as much pain.

One drawback to the Clinitron bed was we couldn't move Howdy out on the front porch during the nice summer weather. He always enjoyed sitting out there watching the people go by. Of course, I didn't spend much time out there either, as I had to be close to Howdy. I wondered why Howdy didn't sweat as much that summer as he used to during the hot weather.

Whenever Howdy was awake, I always tried to make him laugh. I was constantly thinking of funny things to say that'd get a chuckle out of him. It made me feel better when I thought of him having happy thoughts. I felt as if the laughter stimulated him, and his reaction to our laughter pleased us. Because he was sleeping so much, I found myself checking up on him more often to make sure he was still breathing.

How many times can you say, "I love you!" without it becoming too repetitious? Hundreds of times - I know. Even though Howdy was sleeping much more, somehow, I knew he heard me tell him, "I love you!"

I suspected the motion of the bed might've had something to do with Howdy sleeping more, but I wasn't sure. The bed was very sensitive to any movement, so one day I got in and found the bed to be very soothing. Of course there wasn't any "splish-splash," but it was similar to the feeling you get on a waterbed.

Since we didn't belong to any groups or clubs, and we primarily socialized with our son John and his family, we never made lasting friendships like we did in Florida. I was content to devote all of my time to Howdy. We had so many wonderful friends in Florida my memories of the good times we all had together were enough for me to dwell on. Whenever I needed a "mental health break," I was able to drift back to those happy times until I became lost in those memories.

As the summer drew to a close, and we moved into September, we had ample reason to be happy because our grandson, John Howard, was getting married. He, and his bride-to-be, chose September 4th as their wedding day in her home town of Wooster, Ohio. Wooster is a small city in northeast Ohio about an hour-and-a-half drive from where we lived and where John Howard had attended The College of Wooster. After the wedding, they were planning on honeymooning in the Caribbean. The joy we all felt was, of course, tempered by the fact Howdy was desperately hanging on at that time. It seemed any day could be his last, because his breathing became so labored at times it just didn't seem he could survive another setback in his frail condition.

Mary Jane, Jess, their granddaughter Karen, and her boyfriend, Eric, came up to stay with us the night before the wedding. We were going up to Wooster in two cars. When we left on the morning of the 4th, Mary Jane came with me, and the kids followed us.

I only agreed to go if Jess would stay with Howdy while we were gone. I would've really regretted missing my only grandson's wedding, plus it was a chance for me to be with other members of our family for a while. But we knew we'd be gone at least eight hours, and being away from Howdy that long was worrisome for me. Jess agreed to stay with Howdy because he wasn't too keen on going to the wedding and meeting a lot of people he didn't know. Since he knew the routine, and was quite capable of taking care of Howdy, I felt comfortable enough to leave Howdy in Jess' care.

For several days before the wedding, Howdy was very sick. He seemed extremely listless, and didn't have the same glow in his eyes he normally had. I thought his eyes were droopy looking. Given Howdy's condition, it was a very difficult decision for me to go and leave him for such a long time, but our family convinced me I should go, so I did.

It seemed as if we were gone for days instead of only eight hours. Even though we enjoyed the wedding, we were all so glad to get started for home. Howdy was on my mind the whole time we were gone. Once again, I drove with Mary Jane as my passenger, and Karen and Eric followed along behind us. The closer we got to Delaware the more I pushed down on the gas pedal. I didn't realize it at the time, but I was driving faster and faster. Right after exiting I-71 onto routes 36-37 toward Delaware, Mary Jane and I were laughing and talking about the people at the wedding, and having a good conversation. When we first turned onto 36-37, there was a short section of road where the speed limit was 45 mph. We were busy gabbing, so we were zipping right along. All of a sudden, I looked in my rear view mirror and noticed the kids were getting farther and farther behind. I told Mary Jane they were slowing down and wondered why. Just as I started to slow down, I noticed the flashing lights in my rear view mirror. My first thought was, "I wonder who the police are after?" It finally hit me like a ton of bricks. I was the culprit! I pulled to the side of the road, and the patrolman came up to my window and asked for my driver's license. He told me I'd been driving 80 mph in a 45-mph zone. I was shocked, and very nervous. In all the years I'd been driving, that was the first time I'd ever been stopped by a patrolman!

When we left the house that morning, I took what I thought I'd need for the day out of my big purse, and shoved it all into a little purse that went with the outfit I was wearing. I was in a hurry, so I just jammed what I could into the little purse, and I wasn't even sure what all I put in there. With the police officer standing there, I found myself frantically searching through the contents of that little purse, while trying to explain to the officer about Howdy and why we were in such a hurry to get home. Total panic set in when I couldn't find my driver's license! If I said to the officer once, I must have said six times, "You've got to be kidding." I was like a broken record. I really panicked when I dumped out the contents of my purse and the officer saw all the cash I'd taken with me tumble out into my lap. The first thought that went through my mind was he probably thought we were drug dealers. I had visions of Mary Jane and me spending the night at the police station pleading our case. Finally, the officer had to point out to me where the driver's license was in the midst of that mess. Of course, it was right there in plain sight. I thanked God I had it with me. I was so relieved the officer spotted it.

Throughout the entire ordeal, Mary Jane sat right beside me never saying a word. She might as well have been a mummy sitting there. So I had to do all the talking, and boy did I talk! I told him about the wedding and showed him the wedding cake on the floor behind the driver's seat. I must have sounded sincere, or maybe it was just I didn't have any marks against my driving record, but he didn't give me a ticket - just a warning.

For a long time afterward, that incident was good for some laughs in our family. The reason the kids slowed down, of course, was they saw the police car pull out after me. Probably, if it'd been those young kids in the front car, they would've ended up with a ticket. We all had a good laugh about my brush with the law before we went to bed that night. We never knew what was in store for us the next morning - the blackest day of my life.

Because Howdy seemed to be resting a little easier when we got home, we had a fairly good night. The next morning one of the nurses came early to check on Howdy. She never told us Howdy was going downhill. After she checked on him, she went back to the hospital.

At about seven o'clock, Mary Jane went over to see how Howdy was doing. She sounded a little panicky when she called me over to see him.

"Something's wrong!" she said.

The first thing I noticed was how very limp he was - his whole body. That just wasn't normal. He'd been stiff for so long I couldn't understand how he could suddenly become so limp. He felt like a rag doll. He'd been in a fetal position for such a long time it was a shock to see even his legs had straightened a little bit.

From that point on, things went so fast we didn't have time to think. Suddenly, he didn't seem to be breathing. Then he took a big gulp of air. Then nothing. Then another gasp. I was so scared, but I grabbed him in my arms and said, "Don't fight it Howdy, go see your mother and the baby." I was holding him so tight. Then he took one last gulp of air - then nothing. The whole world seemed to collapse before my eyes. I just didn't want to believe he was gone. I was so thankful he went much easier than I thought he'd go, but that still didn't ease the pain of losing him.

For years, I speculated on how he'd die, expecting an agonizing death. I was so relieved he died peacefully. Again, I had to thank God. We were all with him at the end - Mary Jane, Jess, John, and I. At least my grandson didn't have to remember his grandfather died on his wedding day.

Immediately, we called the nurse back. She told us she knew Howdy was failing, but she didn't think it'd be so soon. For a while, I blamed myself for going to the wedding, but I finally got over that.

The house seemed deserted after Howdy was gone. We knew that day was inevitable, but it was still a shock. My mind was filled with many thoughts about Howdy, and about all the things I'd miss about him. I missed the one-sided talks Howdy and I had every day. I missed seeing him lying on that bed and knowing he was getting the best care we could give him. But most of all, I missed just being with him and loving him with all my heart and soul. I had a total feeling of loss that day and for a long time thereafter. How can you explain the terrible, empty, hollow feeling in your heart? How can someone's death be so painful, when you've been taught since childhood there's a much better place for him now? Why do we fear death? With all of the teachings about life after death, why don't we rejoice because our loved one is in heaven where there's no pain, no hate, just love? Even though I was taught about the hereafter and how wonderful it is, I guess I still had my doubts.

You'd think after all of Howdy's suffering, and the way in which we agonized over his deteriorating condition, I'd have had a feeling of relief. But I really didn't. Maybe I would at some point in the future, but not then.

In time, I did come to realize Howdy was better off being with his family and our daughter, so I kept picturing him with his lovable grin and a look of serenity on his face. Those thoughts really helped me get through those difficult times.

I thought I'd cried all of the tears I had in me while nursing Howdy, but the tears kept coming and coming. For many weeks afterward, and for no apparent reason, I'd burst into uncontrollable sobbing, and the memories would come pouring through.

Because of Howdy, I think I became a much better person than I ever hoped to be. So, saying goodbye to my best friend, companion, and lover was the most difficult thing I've ever had to do in my life.

Trying to deal with the necessary details of daily life was unbelievably hard over the weeks and months following Howdy's passing. Disposing of things was the worst part. We decided to do it right away. We had the

Clinitron bed taken away on Monday. We had one of the girls who'd taken care of Howdy come and take all of the medical supplies. She took bed linens, draw sheets, skin lotions, bandages, and just about everything else we used on Howdy. She appreciated having them because she took care of some poor people who needed the supplies, but couldn't afford them. She even took the ointments and non-prescription medicines other people could use. It took her two days to get everything out, and it took us several more days to turn the hospital room back into a living room. The last things to go were Howdy's teeth. I kept them for several years before I could finally part with them. In time, I also gave away all his clothes. The routine of taking care of him, day in and day out, for all those years was extremely hard to get over. The memories are still there; I'll never lose them.

I know I'll see Howdy again. And when that time comes, he'll take me in his arms, stroke my hair, tell me how much he missed me, and how much he still loves me. I'm looking forward to that day with all my heart and soul.

If I had to do it all over again, would I? Oh, yes – gladly!

POST SCRIPT

On January 31, 2009, my mother, Ruth C. Weidman, succumbed to heart failure and passed away at the age of 87. In the years after Howdy passed away, Mom lived a useful and productive life. She managed to accomplish a great deal over the last few years of her life including receiving awards for her paintings, writing this book, and seeing three of her great grandchildren born. Because of her caring nature, infectious sense of humor, and lovable personality, Mom was dearly loved by her entire extended family and many friends, all of whom remember her with loving fondness. Mom truly managed to touch the lives of everyone she met, and we're all better human beings for the joy of having known her. While we all miss her terribly, we know she's now at peace in the House of the Lord, and once again in the arms of her beloved Howdy and holding their child, Barbara Lynn.

John E. Becker

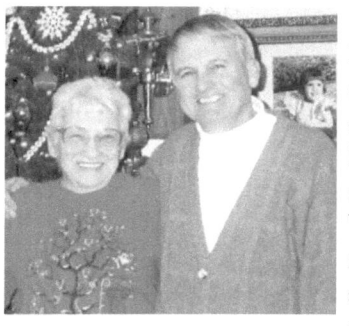

Ruth (Rusty) Zeller was born in Pittsburgh, Pennsylvania in 1921. She moved to Detroit during World War II where she worked at an airplane factory, and then returned to her hometown where she fell in love with the "true love of her life," Howard (Howdy) Weidman. Rusty's life with Howdy over the next four decades was as idyllic a love affair as two people could ever imagine. When they retired to Florida in 1981, Rusty lived a blissful retirement until Howdy began showing signs of Alzheimer's disease in 1983. From that point on, Rusty observed Howdy exhibiting increasingly bizarre behaviors, but her devotion to her husband never wavered as she served as his primary caregiver until he passed away in 1993. Throughout the long ordeal, Rusty had the presence of mind to keep notes of Howdy's daily struggles as he gradually lost his battle with the disease. *Where Did Howdy Go?* is her first book.

Dr. John E. Becker is an award-winning author of 28 books and numerous magazine articles. He coauthored a college textbook, Perceptual Motor Learning Theory and Practice in 1974. His nonfiction children's book, Wild Cats Past & Present, was named to VOYA's (Voice of Youth Advocates) Nonfiction Honor List in the year 2009. Dr. Becker's other books for children include Frenemies for Life, Mugambi's Journey, the fifteen book Returning Wildlife series, and eight Seedling books for beginning readers. Dr. Becker is a graduate of The Ohio State University, a former elementary school teacher, college professor, administrator at the Columbus Zoo, and he worked for many years in the field of wildlife conservation. Dr. Becker is a full-time author living in Delaware, Ohio, and he also teaches writing at the Thurber Writing Academy in Columbus, Ohio. All of his books are listed on his website at www.johnbeckerauthor.com.